CHEMOTHERAPY
HANDBOOK

CHEMOTHERAPY HANDBOOK

Springhouse Corporation
Springhouse, Pennsylvania

Staff

Executive Director, Editorial

Stanley Loeb

Publisher

Barbara F. McVan, RN

Editorial Director

Helen Klusek Hamilton

Art Director

John Hubbard

Drug Information Editor

George J. Blake, RPh, MS

Editors

Rafaela Ellis, Nancy Priff

Clinical Project Editor

Joan E. Mason, RN, MEd

Copy Editors

Christina P. Ponczek, Mary T. Durkin, Kathryn Marino

Designers

Stephanie Peters (associate art director), Lesley Weissman-Cook (book designer), Lorraine Carbo, Jacklyn Facciolo, Mary Ludwicki, Kaaren Mitchel

Typography

David Kosten (director), Diane Paluba (manager), Elizabeth Bergman, Joyce Rossi Biletz, Phyllis Marron, Robin Mayer, Valerie Rosenberger

Manufacturing

Deborah Meiris (director), Anna Brindisi, Kate Davis, T.A. Landis

Production Coordinator

Margaret A. Rastiello

Editorial Assistants

Maree DeRosa, Mary Madden

© 1994 by Springhouse Corporation. All rights reserved. No part of this book may be used or reproduced in any manner whatsoever without written permission except for brief quotations embodied in critical articles and reviews. Printed in the United States of America. For information, write Springhouse Corporation, 1111 Bethlehem Pike, P.O. Box 908, Springhouse, PA 19477-0908.

ISBN 0-87434-618-5

CH-020795

Library of Congress Cataloging-in-Publication Data

Chemotherapy handbook.
  p. cm.
  Includes index.
  1. Drugs – Handbook, manuals,
etc. 2. Chemotherapy – Handbooks, manuals,
etc. 3. Nursing – Handbooks, manuals, etc.
  I. Springhouse Corporation.
  [DNLM: 1. Drug Therapy – handbooks.
  2. Drug Therapy – nurses; instruction. WB 39 C517
1994]
RM301.12.C44   1994
615.5'8–dc20   93-31112
DNLM/DIC   CIP

Contents

Contributors, consultants, and reviewers

Mary Ann Cali-Ascani, RN,C, MSN, OCN
Oncology Nurse Manager, Easton Hospital, Easton, Pa.

Bruce A. Campbell, MD, PhD
Scripps Memorial Hospital, La Jolla, Calif.

James R. Hildebrand, III, PharmD
Director, Drug Information Center, Associate
Professor of Clinical Pharmacy, Philadelphia College
of Pharmacy and Science

Rosaline R. Joseph, MD
Professor of Medicine; Director, Department of
Hematology-Oncology, Medical College of
Pennsylvania, Philadelphia

Mary Jane McDevitt, RN, BS
Staff Nurse, Oncology Unit, Fitzgerald Mercy Division,
Mercy Catholic Medical Center, Darby, Pa.

John J. O'Shea, MD
Expert, Cell Biology and Metabolism, National Institute
of Child Health and Human Development, National
Institutes of Health, Bethesda, Md.

Nancy L. Peck, RN, MSN, CRNI
Nursing Care Coordinator, Thomas Jefferson
University Hospital, Philadelphia

How to use this book

A collaborative effort by physicians, nurses, and pharmacists, *Chemotherapy Handbook* provides comprehensive information on virtually all the drugs administered to combat cancer. It covers all aspects of drug information from fundamental pharmacology to management of extravasation.

An introductory chapter discusses how chemotherapeutic drugs affect the cell cycle, provides guidelines for safe handling of cytotoxic agents, and reviews administration routes and the potential complications of each route.

Drug information

Chapters 2 through 7 contain drug entries. Each of these chapters begins with an alphabetical list of its generic drugs, provides the *pharmacology* of the drug class, gives *clinical indications and actions* and an *overview of adverse reactions*, and concludes with *special considerations* that address patient care and teaching.

In each drug entry, the generic name (with alternate generic names in parentheses) is followed by an alphabetical list of trade names. An asterisk identifies products available only in Canada.

Each drug has been assigned a *Pregnancy risk category* (A, B, C, D, and X) designed by the Food and Drug Administration to reflect a drug's potential to cause birth defects.

A: Adequate studies in pregnant women have failed to show a risk to the fetus in the first trimester of pregnancy — and no evidence suggests a risk in later trimesters.

B: Animal studies have not shown a risk to the fetus, but no adequate clinical studies have been conducted on pregnant women; or animal studies have shown adverse effects on the fetus, but adequate studies in pregnant women have not shown a risk to the fetus during the first trimester of pregnancy, and no evidence suggests a risk in later trimesters.

C: Animal studies have shown an adverse effect on the fetus, but no adequate studies have been conducted on humans; the benefits from use in pregnant women may be acceptable despite potential risks. Or no animal reproduction studies or adequate human studies have been conducted. Therefore, the pregnancy risk is unknown.

D: Studies have shown or suggested some risk to the human fetus, but the potential benefits of use in pregnant women may nonetheless be acceptable.

X: Studies in animals and humans have shown fetal abnormalities, or adverse reaction reports have indicated fetal risk. The risks involved clearly outweigh the potential benefits.

NR: Not rated.

How supplied lists the preparations available for each drug (for example, tablets, capsules, injections, and solutions), specifying dosage forms and strengths. If the drug is available under an investigational protocol, this information and where the drug can be obtained are listed.

Indications, route, and dosage includes weight-specific or body-surface area–specific dosage recommendations. Any off-label uses are indicated by a dagger. These recommendations reflect current clinical use as reported by specialists but cannot be considered absolute or universal.

Pharmacodynamics covers the specific mechanism of action of the drug; *pharmacokinetics* specifies the absorption, distribution, metabolism, and excretion routes, and includes onset and duration of action and half-life when the information is available.

Contraindications and precautions lists conditions associated with special risks in patients who receive the drug and includes the rationale for each warning.

Interactions specifies the clinically significant additive, synergistic, or antagonistic effects that result from drug combinations.

Effects on diagnostic tests lists significant interference with a test or its results by direct effect or by systemic consequences that might alter the results.

Adverse reactions lists recorded undesirable effects. These are arranged by body system (CNS, CV, DERM, EENT, GI, GU, HEMA, Hepatic, Metabolic, Respiratory, Local, and Other). Local effects occur at the site (by application, infusion, or injection); adverse reactions not specific to a single body system (such as hypersensitivity) are listed under Other. Life-threatening reactions are italicized.

Overdose and treatment identifies the clinical manifestations of drug overdose and provides appropriate treatment.

Special considerations offers detailed recommendations for drug preparation and administration, storage, prevention and treatment of adverse reactions, monitoring drug effects, and use in children or breast-feeding patients. (General guidelines are given in the class entry at the beginning of the chapter.) *Information for the patient* follows as a subsection of special considerations. When appropriate, *geriatric use* appears as a second subsection.

Investigational drugs
Chapter 8 addresses drugs that are administered under investigational protocols. Subsections vary depending on the amount of available information. *Pharmacokinetics, interactions*, and *effects on diagnostic tests* are omitted when such data have not been reported.

Pharmacologic management of adverse reactions
This special chapter explores the adverse effects that can be managed by drug therapy — in particular, emesis, stomatitis, and extravasation. Handy charts help identify which drugs have the greatest potential for causing these reactions; specific treatment recommendations are included.

Appendices
These include a list of abbreviations used in this book; a 21-page chart of chemotherapy protocols and acronyms to help sort out the commonly used combination therapies; nomograms for estimating body-surface area in adults and children — essential for determining accurate drug dosages; formulas for calculating body surface area in the adult patient and in the adult patient who is an amputee; and teaching aids to photocopy and give to patients.

Index
The index lists all the drugs by trade and generic names.

Chemotherapy and cancer treatment

Now a mainstay of cancer treatment, chemotherapy has improved care for many patients with formerly untreatable cancers. Chemotherapy is most effective against rapidly growing cancers (leukemia and lymphoma, for example) and less effective against slower growing cancers (such as GI and pulmonary tumors), which have fewer dividing cells at any given moment.

Chemotherapeutic drugs now include more than 50 agents, classified into the following pharmacologic groups:
- alkylating agents
- antibiotic antineoplastics
- antimetabolites
- antineoplastics that alter hormone balance
- biological response modifiers
- miscellaneous antineoplastics

USE IN CANCER

Given alone or in various combinations, chemotherapeutic drugs can inhibit cancer cell growth, prevent metastasis, or relieve symptoms. Chemotherapy given before surgery or radiation therapy, called neoadjuvant or induction or synchronous chemotherapy, can reduce the size of a tumor and improve the surgery's odds for success.

Because chemotherapeutic drugs attack both normal and malignant cells, the challenge of chemotherapy is to provide a dose large enough to destroy the greatest number of cancer cells, but small enough to avoid toxicity or extensive damage to normal tissue. This often can be accomplished by prescribing smaller, concomitant doses of different drugs, which together may be more effective and less toxic than large doses of any single drug. The patient's overall condition and the cancer's stage determine drug selection. However, because cancer cells respond best to the first dose of chemotherapy, doctors strive to select the potentially most effective drugs for the first round of chemotherapy.

To understand how chemotherapeutic drugs work, you must understand cellular kinetics—the study of the growth patterns of normal and malignant cells.

Cell cycle

Normal and malignant cells pass through similar life phases. The first is the G_1 (GAP1) phase, during which active ribonucleic acid (RNA) and protein syntheses take place. Next, the cell moves into the S (synthesis) phase, in which it produces deoxyribonucleic acid (DNA). During this phase, which constitutes one-third to one-half of the total cell cycle, cells are particularly sensitive to many chemotherapeutic drugs.

During the next phase, known as G_2 (GAP2), the cell continues to produce DNA and begins assembling the mitotic spindle apparatus and synthesizing more RNA and protein. Then, the cell divides, or enters the M (mitosis) phase. Some experts believe the divided cell then enters a long resting state, called the G_0 phase.

Some drugs, called cell-cycle specific, are effective only during a specific phase of the cell cycle. Other drugs, called cell-cycle nonspecific, have a prolonged action independent of the cell cycle. (See *How chemotherapeutic drugs disrupt the cell cycle.*)

Where drugs work in the cell cycle

Alkylating agents inhibit cell growth by cross-linking DNA strands. Antibiotic antineoplastics disrupt cell func-

How chemotherapeutic drugs disrupt the cell cycle

Chemotherapeutic drugs may be either cell-cycle specific or cell-cycle non-specific. Cycle-specific drugs, such as methotrexate, act during one or more cell-cycle phases. Cycle-nonspecific drugs, such as busulfan, can act on both replicating and resting cells. (Other examples of cycle-specific agents are listed below.)

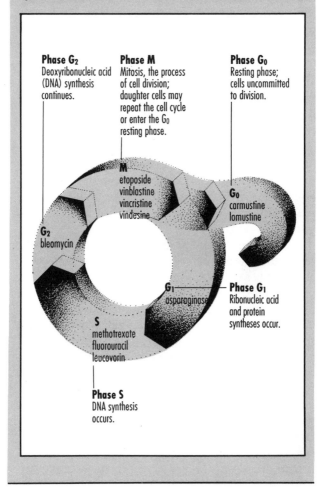

Phase G_2
Deoxyribonucleic acid (DNA) synthesis continues.

Phase M
Mitosis, the process of cell division; daughter cells may repeat the cell cycle or enter the G_0 resting phase.

Phase G_0
Resting phase; cells uncommitted to division.

M
etoposide
vinblastine
vincristine
vindesine

G_0
carmustine
lomustine

G_2
bleomycin

G_1
asparaginase

Phase G_1
Ribonucleic acid and protein syntheses occur.

S
methotrexate
fluorouracil
leucovorin

Phase S
DNA synthesis occurs.

tion by inhibiting RNA and DNA synthesis. Antimetabolites interfere with RNA and DNA synthesis by blocking metabolic pathways or by replacing certain essential metabolites. Antineoplastics that alter hormone balance change the tumor's hormonal environment through various physiologic mechanisms. Biological response modifiers act against tumors by modulating the immune response—for example, by enhancing lymphocyte cytotoxicity. Miscellaneous agents, including plant derivatives and enzymes, exert various cytotoxic effects.

Tumor response

Because a tumor consists of cells at varying stages of the cell cycle, antineoplastic chemotherapy typically uses several drugs to target different cellular sites or different cell-cycle phases. During a single administration of an antineoplastic, a fixed percentage of cells—both normal and malignant—die. Afterward, the remaining cells (again, both normal and malignant) reproduce. Cells that were in the resting phase during chemotherapy may again reproduce.

Therefore, repeated drug doses—spaced at certain intervals to allow normal cell regeneration—are necessary to eradicate a tumor. Commonly, at least three treatments are required before any beneficial response occurs.

Evaluating chemotherapy's effectiveness can be difficult because undetectable cancer cells may survive. Therefore, doctors continue to prescribe chemotherapy even when the patient's cancer seems to be under control.

How well a tumor responds to chemotherapy depends on the percentage of cells killed, the rate of regrowth, the development of resistant cells, and the size of the tumor. Generally, small tumors respond to drugs that affect DNA synthesis, especially cycle-specific drugs; large tumors, on the other hand, respond better to cycle-non-specific drugs.

In advanced or resistant cancers, chemotherapy may be continued as long as the patient can tolerate it without signs of toxicity.

GUIDELINES FOR HANDLING CHEMOTHERAPEUTIC DRUGS

Those who prepare and handle chemotherapeutic drugs face a significant risk. Although the extent of risk hasn't been fully determined, antineoplastics increase the handler's risk of reproductive abnormalities and may also cause hematologic problems. Chronic exposure to them may damage the liver and chromosomes, and direct exposure may burn and damage the skin. These drugs also pose certain environmental dangers. Therefore, care should be taken whenever handling chemotherapeutic drugs.

The Occupational Safety and Health Administration (OSHA) has set guidelines to help ensure the safety of both the handler and the environment. These guidelines include two basic requirements: first, all health care workers who handle chemotherapeutic drugs should be specifically trained for this task, with an emphasis on reducing exposure while handling these drugs; and second, the drugs must be prepared within a Class II biological safety cabinet.

Safety equipment

To protect yourself and the environment, wear a long-sleeved gown, latex surgical gloves, and a face shield or goggles. Make sure you have eyewash, a plastic absorbent pad, alcohol wipes, sterile gauze pads, shoe covers, and an impervious container with the label CAUTION: BIOHAZARD for the disposal of any unused drug or equipment.

Also keep a chemotherapeutic spill kit available. To create a kit, you need a water-resistant, nonpermeable, long-sleeved gown with cuffs and back closure; shoe covers; two pairs of high-grade, extra thick latex gloves (for double-gloving); goggles; a mask; a disposable dustpan and a plastic scraper (for collecting broken glass); plastic-lined or absorbent towels; a container of desiccant powder or granules (to absorb wet contents); two disposable sponges; a puncture-proof, leakproof container labeled

BIOHAZARD WASTE; and a container of 70% isopropyl alcohol for cleaning the spill area.

Precautions for drug preparation

Prepare the prescribed chemotherapeutic drugs according to current product instructions, and with attention to compatibility, stability, and reconstitution technique.

Wash your hands before and after drug preparation and administration. Prepare the drugs in a Class II biological safety cabinet. Wear protective garments, including gloves, as required by the facility's policy. Don't wear these garments outside the preparation area. Never eat, drink, smoke, or apply cosmetics in the drug preparation area.

Before and after preparing the drug, clean the inside of the cabinet with 70% isopropyl alcohol and a disposable towel, which you should discard in a leakproof chemical waste container. Then cover the work surface with a clean, plastic absorbent pad to minimize contamination by droplets or spills. Change the pad at the end of each shift and after any spill.

All drug preparation equipment and any unused drug are hazardous waste. Dispose of them according to the facility's policy. Place all chemotherapeutic waste products in leakproof, sealable, plastic bags or another suitable container, and make sure the container is appropriately labeled.

Special considerations

Reduce exposure to chemotherapeutic drugs by following these guidelines:
- Remember that systemic absorption can occur through ingestion of contaminated materials, contact with the skin, or inhalation. You can accidentally inhale a drug while opening a vial, clipping a needle, expelling air from a syringe, or discarding excess drug that splashes. Drug absorption also can result from handling contaminated feces or body fluids.

- Mix all chemotherapeutic drugs in an approved, Class II biological safety cabinet. Prime all I.V. bags containing these drugs under such a cabinet, and leave the blower on 24 hours a day, 7 days a week. If the safety cabinet doesn't have a hood, prepare drugs in a quiet, well-ventilated work space, away from heating or cooling vents and other personnel.
- Have the biological safety cabinet examined every 6 months, and whenever it is moved, by a company specializing in certifying such equipment.
- Vent vials with a hydrophobic filter, or use negative-pressure techniques. Use a needle with a hydrophobic filter to remove the solution from vials. Break ampules by wrapping a sterile gauze pad or alcohol wipe around the ampule's neck to decrease the chances of droplet contamination.
- Use only syringes and I.V. sets with luer-lock fittings. Mark all chemotherapeutic drugs with CHEMOTHERAPY HAZARD labels.
- Don't clip needles, break syringes, or remove needles from syringes used in drug preparation. Use a gauze pad when removing syringes and needles from I.V. bags of chemotherapeutic drugs.
- Place used syringes, needles, and other sharp or breakable items in a puncture-proof container.
- Change gloves every 30 minutes and whenever you spill a drug solution or puncture or tear a glove. Wash your hands before donning new gloves and anytime you remove your gloves.
- If the drug contacts your skin, wash the area thoroughly with soap (not a germicidal agent) and water. If eye contact occurs, hold open the eyelid and flood the eye with water or isotonic eyewash for at least 5 minutes. Obtain a medical evaluation as soon as possible after accidental exposure.
- Use a chemotherapeutic spill kit to clean up a major spill.
- Discard disposable gowns and gloves in an appropriately marked, waterproof receptacle whenever they be-

come contaminated or whenever you leave the work area.
- Never place food or drinks in a refrigerator that contains chemotherapeutic drugs.
- Understand drug excretion patterns and take appropriate precautions when handling a chemotherapy patient's body fluids.
- Wear disposable latex surgical gloves when handling body fluids or soiled linens. Provide male patients with a urinal with a tight-fitting lid. Before flushing the toilet, place a waterproof pad over the toilet bowl to prevent splashing. Place soiled linens in designated isolation linen bags.
- Remember that women who are pregnant, trying to conceive, or breast-feeding should exercise extreme caution when handling chemotherapeutic drugs.
- Document each exposure incident according to the health care facility's policy.

Home care considerations
Remember these guidelines when administering chemotherapy to a patient at home:
- Expect the patient to obtain the chemotherapeutic drugs from a hospital pharmacy or a specialized retail pharmacy. Expect drugs to be packaged in a sealed plastic bag.
- Before starting chemotherapy, check the patient's insurance to make sure home administration is a covered expense. Remember that if chemotherapy requires a 24-hour continuous infusion, it's typically administered through a portable infusion pump; shorter infusions are commonly given through an implanted port.
- Teach the patient or caregiver to wear two pairs of latex gloves whenever handling chemotherapy equipment, contaminated linens or bedclothes, or body fluids.
- Instruct the patient or caregiver to place soiled linens in a separate washable pillowcase and to launder the pillowcase twice, with the soiled linen inside, separate from other household items.

- Advise the patient or caregiver to arrange for pickup and proper disposal of contaminated waste.
- Tell the patient or caregiver to place all treatment equipment in a leakproof container before disposal.
- Advise the patient or caregiver to dispose of waste products in the toilet, emptying the container close to the water, to minimize splashing. Advise them to close the lid and flush two or three times.

GENERAL GUIDELINES

Chemotherapeutic drugs require careful administration. Some drugs need specialized equipment or unusual administration techniques, while others may become unstable or must be protected from light. Most important, the dosage of these potent drugs must be precise to avoid possibly fatal complications. Therefore, only specially trained nurses and doctors should administer chemotherapeutic drugs.

Routes

Chemotherapeutic drugs are most commonly administered I.V. through a peripheral vein or a central venous line—for example, by a Hickman catheter, a vascular access port (also called a vascular access device), or a peripherally inserted central catheter or midline catheter. The drugs may also be given orally, subcutaneously, or intramuscularly; through a reservoir into the spinal canal; or into an artery, the peritoneal cavity, or the pleural space.

The route selected depends on several factors, including the character of the tumor, the drug's pharmacodynamics, the prescribed dosage, the patient's overall health (including vascular status), his lifestyle, the available resources, and most effective method of administration.

Dosage

Although higher doses of chemotherapeutic drugs usually prove more effective than lower doses, adverse drug ef-

fects often limit the dosage. One exception to this rule is
methotrexate, which is effective against rapidly growing
tumors but toxic to growing and rapidly dividing normal
tissues. Administering leucovorin with a large dose of
methotrexate can preserve normal tissue (see *Leucovorin
rescue*).

Preparation

Before administering a chemotherapeutic drug, assess the
patient's physical condition and review his medical history. Evaluate the patient's and family's desire for information and their level of understanding, and correct any
misconceptions about the disease or treatments. Teach
specifically about the prescribed chemotherapeutic drug,
the treatment protocol, and the administration schedule.
Reassure the patient that pain can be managed, and discuss the potential adverse effects of chemotherapy. Understand which drugs will be given and by what route, and
provide teaching and support to the patient and family.

When evaluating the patient's condition, pay particular attention to the results of recent laboratory studies,
specifically CBC, BUN, platelet count, urine creatinine
level, and liver function studies.

Review the patient's medical history for previous chemotherapy, noting the severity of any adverse effects, and
check the patient's medication history for drugs that
might interact with chemotherapy. As a rule, don't mix
chemotherapeutic drugs with any other medications. If
you have questions or concerns about administering chemotherapeutic drugs, discuss them beforehand with the
pharmacist or the patient's doctor.

Next, double-check the chart for the chemotherapy
protocol order, including the patient's name, the drug's
name and dose, and the route, rate, and frequency of administration. Determine if the dosage depends on certain
laboratory values. Some health care facilities require that
two nurses read the dosage order, check the drug and the
amount being administered, and review laboratory
results.

Leucovorin rescue

Methotrexate interferes with cell division in the cell cycle's S phase by inhibiting dihydrofolate reductase, an enzyme involved in DNA synthesis. (See *How chemotherapeutic drugs disrupt the cell cycle*, page 3.) High-dose methotrexate therapy is most effective against cells with a high metabolic rate, such as leukemia cells. Used alone, high doses of methotrexate eventually affect normal cells as well.

To protect normal cells, methotrexate is commonly prescribed with leucovorin (folinic acid). Leucovorin rescues cells by bypassing the S phase. To work efficiently, it must be administered exactly as prescribed—with proper doses given at the proper times and without skipping doses. When given correctly, leucovorin rescues cells before they begin active growth and division.

Because leucovorin can't prevent methotrexate toxicity completely, you should monitor the patient on high-dose methotrexate therapy for bone marrow suppression, stomatitis, pulmonary complications, and renal damage (from drug precipitation in the renal tubules). Also maintain the patient's urine alkalinity to avoid drug precipitation, and monitor his urine output.

Verify whether the doctor has ordered administration of an antiemetic, fluids, or a diuretic before chemotherapy, or of electrolyte supplements before, during, or afterward. Finally, talk with the patient and family to evaluate their understanding of chemotherapy, and make sure that the patient, caregiver (an adult if the child is a minor), or the person with durable power of attorney has signed the consent form.

Next, don gloves and keep them on throughout all stages of drug handling—including preparation, priming the I.V. tubing, and administration.

ADMINISTERING CHEMOTHERAPEUTIC DRUGS

Peripheral administration

You may give chemotherapeutic drugs peripherally, using a bolus or continuous infusion. The bolus method delivers a one-time dose; a continuous infusion delivers the necessary dose over a given period.

Before giving the drug, perform a new venipuncture proximal to the old site. Avoid giving chemotherapeutic drugs through an existing peripheral I.V. line. To identify an administration site, examine the patient's veins, beginning with the hand and proceeding to the forearm (see *Peripheral and central veins used in I.V. therapy*).

When selecting a site, consider drug compatibilities, the frequency of administration, and the drug's vesicant potential. (To identify vesicant drugs, see *Determining vesicant potential* in Chapter 9.)

Special considerations

The Oncology Nursing Society has established the following guidelines for the peripheral administration of chemotherapy by bolus or continuous infusion:

- Select the appropriate equipment.
- Have the patient reposition restrictive clothing and jewelry. Reposition his identification bracelet, if necessary.
- Examine the the patient's veins and ask his opinions regarding site selection.
- Proceed from hand to forearm.
- Avoid the site of a previous mastectomy, phlebitis, an invading neoplasm, or hematoma; the antecubital fossa, lower extremities, varicosities, inflamed or sclerosed areas or those with impaired lymphatic drainage or venous circulation; and sites distal to recent venipunctures.
- Alternate arms if possible.
- Avoid using an existing peripheral I.V. line.
- Apply heat if necessary to distend the veins.
- Verify each drug, the dose, and the patient's identification.
- Wash hands.
- Apply a tourniquet.
- Clean the site according to the facility's policy and procedure.

Peripheral and central veins used in I.V. therapy

This illustration shows the veins commonly used for peripheral I.V. and central venous therapy. *Note:* Vesicant drugs should not be given in the antecubital fossa, near the wrist, or the dorsum of the hand.

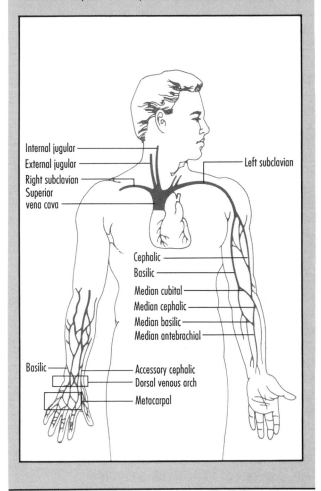

- Insert the needle, observe blood backflow, and remove the tourniquet; tape the needle to allow observation of insertion site.
- Stabilize the hand or arm; use an armboard or pillow if necessary.
- Infuse sterile 0.9% sodium chloride solution or sterile water for injection.
- Observe for infiltration continuously during bolus infusion; observe the site of continuous infusions at least every 30 minutes.
- Administer drugs as ordered according to approved policy of the facility.
- Observe the site for swelling, redness, blebs, or hives.
- Encourage the patient to report such sensations as pain, burning, or stinging.
- Periodically reconfirm vein patency (for example, lower the I.V. bag and observe for blood return, or aspirate until blood return is noted).
- Provide sufficient 0.9% sodium chloride solution or sterile water for injection between drug infusions to completely flush the I.V. lines of residual drugs.
- Monitor the patient for adverse reactions during and after treatment.
- Infuse 0.9% sodium chloride solution or sterile water for injection posttreatment.
- Remove the needle and apply a sterile dressing.
- Elevate the extremity and apply pressure for 3 to 5 minutes. Observe for hematoma after 5 minutes.
- Apply an adhesive strip to the site.
- Dispose of equipment according to the facility's policy.
- Wash hands.
- Document the procedure according to the facility's policy.

Local complications: Treatment and prevention

Peripheral venous therapy can produce both local and systemic complications. Common local complications include phlebitis, extravasation and infiltration, occlusion, venous irritation, severed catheter, hematoma, venous spasm, and thrombosis.

Phlebitis. Phlebitis begins as a redness starting at the catheter tip and continuing up the vein. The patient may complain of tenderness along the catheter and above it. The vein may feel hard, and the surrounding tissue may be edematous and warm.

Possible causes of phlebitis include a clot at the catheter tip, catheter movement within the vessel, poor blood flow around the catheter, a catheter that's left in the vessel too long, or an infused solution with a particularly high or low pH or a high osmolarity.

Treat phlebitis by removing the catheter immediately and applying warm soaks to the affected area. If the patient develops a fever, notify the doctor. To prevent phlebitis, try these measures:
- When inserting a new catheter, use either a larger vein or a smaller-gauge catheter to ensure adequate blood flow.
- Use an in-line filter to eliminate small particles that may cause irritation.
- Securely anchor the venipuncture device to prevent any irritating movement.
- Change the catheter site regularly and at the first sign of vein tenderness or redness.

Extravasation and infiltration. The leakage of a vesicant solution into the surrounding tissues is known as extravasation. Leakage of a nonvesicant solution into the surrounding tissues is infiltration. Signs of these common complications include swelling at and above the I.V. site, decreased skin temperature, blanching around the site, and a slow drip rate. (With an infusion pump, the flow rate may continue despite an occlusion.) The patient may complain of burning, tightness, and pain at the site.

To prevent extravasation, check the I.V. site often, especially if you use an infusion pump. Don't apply tape or tight restraints above the site. Tell the patient to promptly report any discomfort, pain, or swelling.

Partial retraction from the vein or infiltration into the surrounding tissues may also cause these complications.

If so, make sure the I.V. line isn't tangled in the patient's clothes or bed linens. If the I.V. solution hasn't infiltrated, retape the I.V. without pushing the catheter farther into the vein. If the solution has infiltrated, replace the I.V. line with a new one. Make sure the I.V. catheter and tubing are securely taped.

Remember that seeing a blood return in an I.V. catheter doesn't confirm that the catheter is in the vein. Similarly, a lack of blood return doesn't always mean the catheter isn't in the vein.

Occlusion. Two signs indicate occlusion: blood backflow into the I.V. tubing and a flow rate that doesn't increase when the bag is elevated. Occlusion may result from interruption of the I.V. flow rate during a piggyback infusion, from a heparin lock that's not flushed, or from a backflow of blood into the tubing when the patient moves. If you observe an occlusion, aspirate and then flush the I.V. line using mild pressure. If that doesn't work, remove the line and restart it in a new site.

To prevent occlusion, check the I.V. line frequently and maintain the I.V. flow rate. Always flush a heparin lock after you administer each drug. Encourage the patient to avoid a backflow of blood by walking with his arm across his chest.

Venous irritation. During an I.V. infusion, the patient may feel irritation or pain. The site may blanch during a venous spasm, or the skin over the vein may redden. Certain solutions, including potassium chloride, vancomycin, nafcillin, phenytoin, or those with a high or low pH or high osmolarity, also may cause irritation.

Relieve the patient's discomfort by slowing the infusion rate and using an infusion pump to maintain a steady flow. You may dilute the I.V. medication in 250 ml of solution, or check with the doctor and pharmacist to see if the solution can be buffered with sodium bicarbonate. Apply ice or heat over the I.V. site to ease discomfort during the infusion.

Severed catheter. If the catheter leaks solution, it may have been accidentally severed during insertion. If so, and the broken part is visible, try to retrieve it. Otherwise, apply a tourniquet above the I.V. site.

To avoid this problem, never use scissors when inserting a catheter and never reinsert the needle into the catheter. If you're unable to insert the catheter, remove the catheter and needle together.

Hematoma. A hematoma may result if the opposite vein wall is punctured during insertion or if infiltration causes blood leakage into the surrounding tissue. If the patient has a hematoma, you won't be able to advance the catheter beyond a certain point, the patient may complain of tenderness at the insertion site, and you also may notice bruising at the site. If so, remove the catheter and reinsert it at a new site. Apply pressure to the area, and recheck the hematoma site periodically for bleeding. After the bleeding stops, apply warm soaks.

Venous spasm. The patient who complains of pain along the vein may be experiencing venous spasm. If so, the I.V. flow rate will be sluggish even when the roller clamp is fully open. Venous spasm may result from irritant solutions, from the administration of cold medications, and from a rapid infusion rate.

To treat venous spasm, apply warm soaks over the area and slow the infusion rate. To prevent spasm, allow solutions to reach room temperature before infusion.

Thrombosis. A painful, reddened, and swollen vein, along with a sluggish or stopped I.V. flow, indicates thrombosis. This complication results when the vein wall's endothelial cells are injured, allowing platelets to adhere and a thrombus to form.

If you suspect thrombosis, remove the I.V. line immediately and reinsert it in another line, if possible. Apply warm soaks and monitor the site for infection.

Systemic complications: Treatment and prevention
Four systemic complications may result from I.V. therapy: circulatory overload, systemic infection, speed shock,
and allergic reaction.

Circulatory overload. The patient with this life-threatening
condition, typically caused by an increased flow rate over
time, may show signs of CHF, increased blood pressure,
crackles, neck vein distention, and shortness of breath.
  If you suspect circulatory overload, notify the patient's doctor immediately. Raise the head of the patient's
bed; then administer oxygen and medications, as ordered.
To prevent circulatory overload, use a pump when administering I.V. therapy to patients who have problems elimi-
nating fluids (for example, those with a history of CHF,
decreased renal function, and decreased cardiac output).
Check and monitor the flow rate frequently.

Systemic infection. Failure to use aseptic technique, severe
phlebitis, prolonged use of a venipuncture device, and
poor catheter taping that introduces microorganisms into
the vein can cause this complication. The patient with systemic infection has chills, fever, and unexplained malaise.
  Notify the patient's doctor, obtain a culture of the infected site, and give any ordered medications. To prevent
systemic infection, always use aseptic technique when inserting a new catheter. Change sites, tubing, and solutions
when appropriate, and make sure all connections are
secure.

Speed shock. Most common with bolus injections, speed
shock occurs when a drug is administered too quickly,
causing toxic plasma levels. The patient will have a headache, syncope, a flushed face, tightness in his chest, an irregular pulse and, possibly, shock and cardiac arrest.
  If you suspect speed shock, discontinue the infusion
immediately and notify the patient's doctor. You may give
dextrose 5% in water at a keep-vein-open rate. To prevent
speed shock, be sure to follow the manufacturer's recommendations for administering a drug.

Allergic reaction. Restlessness, agitation, itching, broncho-spasm, wheezing, urticaria, and edema at the I.V. site may signal an allergic reaction. If you suspect this complication, stop the infusion immediately and notify the patient's doctor. Help maintain the patient's cardiopulmonary status, and give corticosteroids, NSAIDs, and epinephrine if ordered.

To prevent allergic reactions, record the patient's allergic history and remember that a delayed repeat allergic reaction can occur hours after an initial reaction.

Central venous administration

To facilitate chemotherapy, the doctor may insert a central venous line directly into the patient's subclavian or internal jugular vein. Depending on the catheter type, the line terminates in the superior vena cava. (See *Identifying CV catheter pathways,* page 20.)

Catheters used with central venous lines include the commonly used Hickman catheter and the Broviac or Groshong catheters, used for long-term central venous infusions. Depending on the drug and dosage, a short-term central venous catheter also may be used.

Administering chemotherapy through a central line
Chemotherapy may be administered into a central line by direct push, into an existing line, or in a bolus through the side port of an infusing line (intermittent), or as a continuous infusion.

Bolus dose. To give a bolus dose through a central venous line, gather a syringe with the prescribed drug, alcohol wipes, two 3- to 5-ml syringes with 0.9% sterile sodium chloride solution, and heparin solution. Then proceed as follows:
- Explain the procedure to the patient and don clean gloves.
- Clean the injection cap with an alcohol wipe and flush it with sterile 0.9% sodium chloride solution.

Identifying CV catheter pathways

Usually, a central venous (CV) catheter is inserted into the subclavian vein or the internal jugular vein. The catheter may terminate in the superior vena cava or the right atrium. The illustrations below show several common pathways of the CV catheter.

This CV catheter, inserted into the subclavian vein, terminates in the superior vena cava.

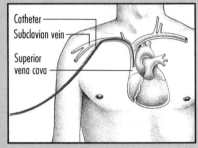

Inserted into the subclavian vein, this CV catheter extends to the right atrium.

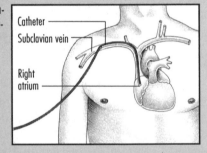

This CV catheter enters the internal jugular vein and terminates in the superior vena cava.

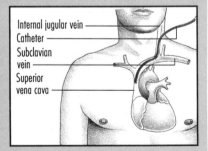

- Insert the needle of the syringe containing the drug, and slowly inject the drug according to the manufacturer's directions or the facility's policy.
- Withdraw the needle and discard it (but don't recap it).
- Clean the injection cap again with an alcohol wipe; then inject the cap with 3 to 5 ml of the sterile sodium chloride solution.
- Clean the cap a third time; then inject it with heparin solution, according to the facility's policy.

Intermittent administration. Chemotherapeutic drugs may be given intermittently through a central venous line (typically over 40 to 60 minutes). You'll either inject a drug into an existing I.V. line that feeds into the central venous line or administer the drug through an injection cap.

If using an injection cap, gather the prescribed drug, I.V. tubing, a short needle (1" or smaller), two 3- to 5-ml syringes filled with sterile 0.9% sodium chloride solution, heparin solution, and alcohol wipes. Attach a needle or appropriate needleless system to the end of the I.V. tubing, according to the facility's policy. Then proceed as follows:

- Explain the procedure to the patient and don clean gloves.
- Clean the top of the injection cap with an alcohol wipe.
- Flush the catheter through the injection cap with 3 to 5 ml of sterile 0.9% sodium chloride solution.
- Plug the needle into the injection cap and start the infusion at the desired rate.
- Tape over the non-luer-lock connections to prevent disconnection.
- When the infusion is complete, close the roller clamp on the I.V. tubing. Unplug the needle and discard it, but don't recap it—this could cause a needle-stick injury.
- Clean the injection cap again and flush with heparin solution, according to the facility's policy. (*Note:* If the patient has a Groshong catheter, flush with 0.9% sodium chloride solution, not heparin.)

Continuous infusion. When administering an I.V. solution by continuous infusion (usually longer than 30 minutes), prepare the solution and tubing. Use a volumetric control device to ensure accurate delivery of the solution. Then follow these guidelines:

- Explain the procedure to the patient and don clean gloves.
- If you plan to attach I.V. tubing to a capped lumen, first flush the lumen with 0.9% sodium chloride solution.
- Clamp the catheter, but only where indicated. If the catheter has neither its own clamp nor a designated clamp location, choose a smooth-edged clamp, or clamp the catheter over some tape. Avoid toothed clamps, which may damage the catheter.
- If no clamp is available, have the patient perform Valsalva's maneuver to help prevent air embolism. As he bears down and takes a deep breath, remove the cap and plug in the I.V. tubing.
- Set the ordered flow rate on the I.V. controller or pump.
- Tape over any non-luer-lock connections to prevent disconnection.

Care considerations

Use the following guidelines when caring for a patient with a central venous line.

Changing the dressing. Change the dressing every 48 to 72 hours or whenever it becomes soiled or nonocclusive. Before you begin, gather the following: clean and sterile gloves, alcohol wipes, povidone-iodine swabs, antiseptic or povidone-iodine ointment, sterile transparent semipermeable dressing, sterile gauze pads, and adhesive tape. To prevent contamination, always use sterile technique and follow the facility's policy.

First, explain the procedure to the patient and don clean gloves. Remove the old dressing, taking care not to dislodge the catheter. Remove and discard the gloves and the dressing.

Next, don sterile gloves, and clean the skin around the site with alcohol wipes or pads soaked in hydrogen peroxide or chlorhexidine gluconate. Start at the center of the site and move outward, using a circular motion. Repeat the cleaning process twice, using a fresh wipe or pad each time. Allow the skin to dry; then repeat the procedure using povidone-iodine swabs.

After the solution has dried, apply a small amount of antiseptic or povidone-iodine ointment to the site, according to the facility's policy. Then secure the catheter to the skin and cover the site with a transparent semipermeable dressing or sterile gauze pads and tape. Label the dressing with the date, time, and your initials.

Changing I.V. tubing and solution. Change I.V. tubing and solutions every 24 hours or as your facility requires. After preparing the new tubing and solution, explain the procedure to the patient, and don clean gloves.

Stop the current infusion and clamp the catheter, using the clamp attached to the catheter or at the catheter's designated clamp location. Do not use a toothed clamp. If no clamp is available, have the patient perform Valsalva's maneuver, if possible.

Replace the old I.V. tubing with new tubing. Set the infusion pump to the prescribed rate, and discard the old solution and tubing.

Changing the injection cap. The injection cap on a central venous catheter used for intermittent infusion should be changed regularly—every 3 to 7 days in most facilities.

Begin by explaining the procedure to the patient and donning clean gloves. Clean the old injection cap with an alcohol wipe at its connection to the catheter. Clamp the catheter at the proper location, or have the patient perform Valsalva's maneuver. Using aseptic technique, remove the old cap and connect the new cap.

Flushing the catheter. Flush a central catheter after every drug or fluid administration and regularly between administrations to keep it patent.

For a short-term catheter, flush with a heparin solution of 10 to 100 units/3 to 5 ml every 12 hours, or according to the manufacturer's recommendations or the facility's policy. For a long-term catheter, flush with a heparin solution of 100 units/5 ml every 12 to 24 hours or longer, depending on the catheter. For a Groshong catheter, flush with 5 ml of sterile 0.9% sodium chloride solution every 7 days. If the patient is receiving a highly viscous fluid, such as with total parenteral nutrition (TPN), or if blood samples have been drawn through the catheter, flush with 20 ml of 0.9% sodium chloride solution to prevent crystallization of the catheter tip.

To flush the catheter, gather alcohol wipes, 3 to 5 ml of sterile 0.9% sodium chloride solution in a syringe, heparin flush solution, and clean gloves. Explain the procedure to the patient. Then don gloves, and clean the injection cap with the alcohol wipe.

Insert the syringe filled with sterile 0.9% sodium chloride solution, and gently flush the catheter. Clean the injection cap again, insert the heparin solution in a syringe, and flush the catheter a second time. As you withdraw the syringe with the flush solution, continue to put pressure on the plunger to prevent blood from entering the catheter.

Complications

Complications can occur at any time during central venous therapy. Traumatic complications such as pneumothorax typically occur during catheter insertion, although they may not be detected until later. Systemic complications, such as sepsis, usually develop after the catheter has been in place for a time. Other complications include air embolism, local infection, cardiac tamponade, thrombus formation, and phlebitis.

Traumatic complications. These complications may result when the catheter punctures a lung, blood vessel, or lymph node during insertion or exchange over the guide wire, or when the infusing solution infiltrates the chest. Traumatic complications typically cause chest pain, dyspnea, cyanosis, decreased breath sounds, abnormal chest X-ray, and reduced hemoglobin (with hemothorax). If these complications occur, notify the patient's doctor, and remove the catheter or assist with removal. Administer oxygen, as ordered. Prepare for and assist with chest tube insertion. Finally, document the procedure. To prevent these complications, follow these guidelines:

- Place the patient in Trendelenburg's position, with a rolled towel between the shoulder blades, to dilate the vein and make it more visible.
- Assess for early signs of fluid infiltration (swelling in shoulder, neck, chest, and arm).
- Immobilize the patient by adequately preparing him for the procedure and restraining him during insertion. An active patient may require sedation or surgical intervention.

Air embolism. Causes of air embolism include air intake into the central venous system during catheter insertion or tubing changes; or inadvertent opening, cutting, or breakage of the catheter. Typical symptoms include respiratory distress, unequal breath sounds, weak pulse, elevated central venous pressure, decreased blood pressure, churning murmur over the precordium, and loss of consciousness.

If air embolism occurs, clamp the catheter immediately. Turn the patient onto his left side, with his head down so that air can enter the right atrium and disperse through the pulmonary artery. Have the patient maintain this position for 20 to 30 minutes. Administer oxygen, as ordered, and notify the patient's doctor. To prevent air embolism, follow these guidelines:

- Purge all air from tubing before hookup.
- Have the patient perform Valsalva's maneuver during catheter insertion and tubing changes.
- Use air-elimination filters proximal to the patient.
- Use an infusion control device with air detection capability.
- Tape all connections or use locking tubing or luer-lock connectors.

Thrombosis. Possible causes of thrombosis include a sluggish flow rate; use of thrombogenic catheter material; preexisting limb edema, abnormal hematopoietic status, or cardiovascular disease; infusion of irritating solutions; or repeated or prolonged use of the same vein.

Typical signs and symptoms include edema at the puncture site; erythema; ipsilateral swelling of the arm, neck, and face; pain along the vein; fever; malaise; and tachycardia.

If thrombosis occurs, notify the patient's doctor, remove the catheter, and infuse anticoagulant doses of heparin, if ordered. Apply warm, wet compresses locally. Do not use the limb on the affected side for venipuncture. Verify thrombosis with diagnostic test results, and document your actions. To prevent thrombosis, follow these guidelines:

- Maintain a steady catheter flow by using an infusion pump or flushing regularly.
- Use a catheter made of less thrombogenic material or one coated to discourage thrombosis (if permitted). Dilute irritating solutions.
- Use a 0.22-micron in-line filter.

Local infection. Failure to maintain aseptic technique during catheter insertion or site care, failure to follow dressing change protocol, presence of a wet or soiled dressing, immunosuppression, or irritation at the suture line may cause local infection.

Signs and symptoms include redness, warmth, tenderness, and swelling at the catheter's insertion or exit site; purulent exudate; local rash or pustules; fever; chills; and malaise.

If local infection develops, monitor the patient's temperature frequently. Culture the site. Redress the site aseptically and apply an antibiotic ointment, as ordered. Treat with systemic antibiotic or antifungal agents, depending on the culture's results and as prescribed. Remove the catheter, as ordered. To prevent local infection, follow these guidelines:

- Maintain strict aseptic technique and follow dressing change protocols.

- Teach the patient about swimming and bathing restrictions.
- Change a wet dressing immediately.
- Change the dressing more frequently if the catheter is in the femoral area or near a tracheostomy.

Systemic infection. Possible causes of systemic infection include a contaminated catheter or infused solution; failure to maintain aseptic technique during solution hookup; frequent opening of the catheter or prolonged use of the access site; and immunosuppression. Signs and symptoms include unexplained fever, chills, elevated WBC count, nausea and vomiting, malaise, and elevated urine glucose level.

If the patient develops a systemic infection, obtain central and peripheral line blood cultures. If results show the same organism, the catheter is the source of sepsis; it should be removed and the tip should be cultured. If the results of the cultures differ but are positive, remove the catheter or treat the infection through the catheter. Administer antibiotics, as ordered. Also assess for other sources of infection. Monitor the patient's vital signs closely. Document the procedure. To prevent systemic infection, follow these guidelines:

- Examine the I. V. fluid container for cloudiness, leaks, and turbidity before infusing.
- Monitor urine glucose levels in patients receiving TPN; suspect early sepsis if the level is greater than 2.
- Use strict aseptic technique for hookup and fluid discontinuation.
- Use a 0.22-micron in-line filter.
- Change the catheter frequently, if necessary, to decrease the risk of infection.
- Avoid unnecessarily manipulating the catheter, and maintain a closed system. Teach other personnel and the patient about the need for aseptic technique.

Cardiac tamponade. This life-threatening complication results when the catheter perforates the heart wall. It causes pulsus paradoxus, jugular vein distention, narrowed pulse pressure, muffled heart sounds, diaphoresis, and dyspnea.

To manage cardiac tamponade, give oxygen and prepare the patient for emergency surgery, as ordered. Monitor the patient continuously, and have emergency equipment available. To prevent cardiac tamponade, follow these guidelines:

- Immobilize the patient during catheter insertion.
- Verify the catheter's position with a chest X-ray.
- Monitor the patient for signs and symptoms of cardiac tamponade.

Vascular access ports

Inserted surgically under local anesthesia, vascular access ports (VAPs), also called vascular access devices (VADs), provide for periodic infusion of chemotherapeutic drugs. A VAP poses a lower risk of infection than a central venous line because it has no exit site to allow entry of microorganisms.

Two basic VAP designs are available: top entry (such as Med-i-port, Port-A-Cath, and Infus-A-Port) and side entry (such as S.E.A. Port). VAPs also are classified as high- or low-profile depending on their height—usually $1/2$" to 1" (1.3 to 2.5 cm). Low-profile VAPs are typically more stable; high-profile VAPs allow easier access.

The VAP reservoir attaches to a 20" to 30" (50.8- to 76.2-cm) radiopaque silicone catheter (a Hickman or Groshong catheter may also be used). Catheter placement is verified by fluoroscopy or X-ray. Other VAPs are available as a single preconnected unit, or as a two-part system that's connected after placement. (See *Vascular access port.*)

VAP insertion. Implantable central venous devices are inserted and removed on an outpatient basis, commonly in the operating room under local anesthesia.

Immediately after insertion, carefully examine the port's pocket incision for hematoma, excess swelling, exudate, thrombosis, port rotation, or port extrusion. Assess the incision for redness, swelling, or drainage related to infection. Expect some tenderness and swelling around

Vascular access port

The large illustration below provides a cutaway view of drug injection through a vascular access port (VAP). The insert shows the entire VAP device.

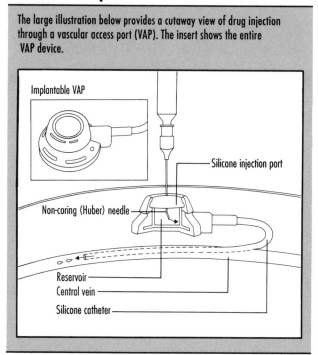

Implantable VAP

Silicone injection port

Non-coring (Huber) needle

Reservoir
Central vein
Silicone catheter

the site for about 72 hours after insertion. No special care is required after the incision heals (usually in 5 to 7 days).

You can use the VAP immediately after insertion unless the site is extremely painful, tender, or swollen, or if the doctor requests radiologic verification of placement. When you're ready to proceed, access the port and give a bolus injection or initiate a continuous infusion, using universal precautions.

Giving a bolus injection. Gather povidone-iodine swabs, a needle and syringe containing 3 to 5 ml of heparin solution (100 units/ml), a 10-ml syringe (with needle) containing sterile 0.9% sodium chloride solution, a non-coring needle, 6" (15-cm) I.V. extension tubing, the prescribed drug, and sterile gloves and mask. Then follow these steps:

- After washing your hands, palpate the port, assessing its depth and size.

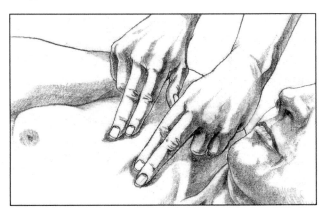

- If you can't palpate a deeply inserted port, use a $^1/_2$" needle to gain access. If the patient fears the needle, numb the port area with an ice pack for 1 or 2 minutes or infiltrate the area with a local anesthetic, such as 0.1 to 0.15 ml of 2% lidocaine solution. If the port has been in place for a long time, confirm its location with a chest X-ray.
- Clean the site with povidone-iodine swabs, according to the facility's policy. Don sterile gloves and a mask. Stabilize the reservoir between your thumb and forefinger. Hold the non-coring needle like a dart, and position it at a 90-degree angle over the septum.

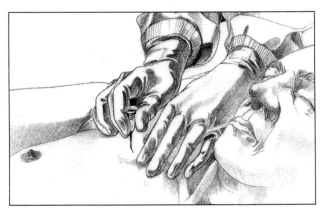

- Push the needle vertically through the skin and septum (not at an angle, which could damage the septum) until it hits the needle stop at the back of the septum. Then, attach the extension tubing to the needle hub.

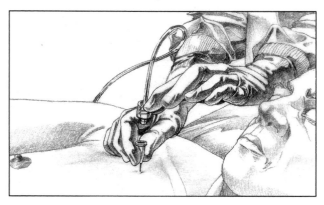

Note: You may also attach a stopcock to the needle hub to maintain a closed system and minimize needle manipulation.

- To check needle placement, aspirate for blood return. If you see no blood return, have the patient cough, turn, raise his arm, or take a deep breath. If this doesn't induce blood return, remove the needle and repeat the procedure at a different site.
- When adequate blood return is established, steadily inject 5 ml of 0.9% sodium chloride flush solution.

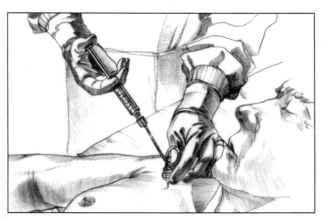

- If you can't inject the solution, the needle tip probably is not positioned correctly. Advance the needle tip to the needle stop and try to inject the solution again. If you fail again, remove the syringe.
- After injecting the flush solution, remove the syringe.

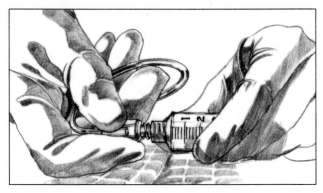

- Next, inject the prescribed drug into the extension tubing port. *Important:* To prevent drug incompatibility, flush the device with 0.9% sodium chloride solution before and after each injection and before each heparin flush. Flush the tubing with 3 to 5 ml of heparin flush solution, according to the facility's policy. *(Note:* During regular use, the port won't need additional heparin flushing; when not in use, flush it monthly to maintain patency.)

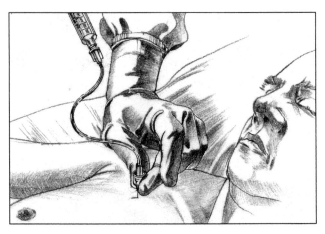

- When the infusion is complete, remove the needle. Stabilize the reservoir between your thumb and forefinger; then withdraw the needle, taking care not to twist or bend it. After needle withdrawal, you may observe a slight serosanguineous discharge at the insertion site.

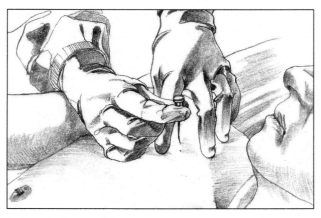

Giving a continuous infusion. To give a continuous infusion, follow these instructions:
- Use extension tubing with a luer-lock and clamp and a right-angle non-coring needle.

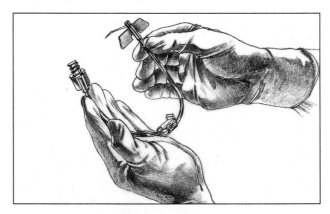

- Remove all air from the extension tubing by priming it with an attached syringe of 0.9% sodium chloride solution. Clean the insertion site and prime the I.V. tubing.

- Using sterile technique, insert the needle and stabilize it at its hub to prevent rotation. The needle's upper portion should lie just above the skin surface; if it's more than 0.5 cm above the surface, support it with a folded 2" × 2" gauze pad.
- Use sterile adhesive strips to secure the needle hub first; then secure the extension tubing.
- Apply povidone-iodine ointment to the insertion site. Then apply a transparent semipermeable dressing.

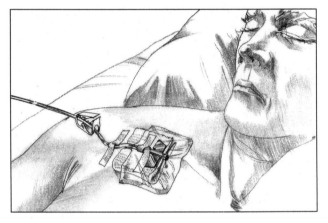

- Connect the I.V. administration set, secure the connection with sterile tape, then unclamp the administration set and begin the infusion. Monitor the site for infiltration. If the patient complains of stinging, burning, or pain, discontinue the infusion and intervene appropriately.
- When the solution container is empty, obtain a new I.V. solution container, as ordered. If the patient is receiving a continuous or prolonged infusion, change the dressing and needle every 3 to 5 days; change the tubing and solution as you would for a long-term central venous infusion.

Complications. A patient with a VAP risks thrombosis, erythema, burning, and catheter blockage. Learn to recognize and manage these complications.

Thrombosis. Inadequate flushing of the system, too-frequent blood sampling, or blood transfusion may cause thrombosis. To detect thrombosis, examine the patient's hand, neck, and shoulder on the side of the port for edema and tenderness. Treatment typically includes fibrinolytic therapy.

Erythema. Excessive patient movement while the needle is in place or repeated use of the same access site may cause erythema. Localized infection may develop, causing redness and drainage at the site. Erythema can lead to systemic infection, with fever, lethargy, and other flulike symptoms.

Treatment typically includes antibiotics and possible removal of the port. If the port is the suspected source of the infection, expect to obtain blood cultures from it. Even if cultures confirm that the port is the infection source, the port can still be used to administer antibiotics.

Blocked catheter. The most common problem associated with VAPs, a blocked catheter can result from kinked tubing, pump malfunction, improper needle or catheter position, port rotation, or port dislodgment.

Straighten kinked tubing, replace a malfunctioning pump, and remove and replace an incorrectly placed needle. Rotation or dislodgment of the port requires the doctor's intervention. If you suspect that the catheter is lodged against the vessel wall, have the patient change position, reaccess the port, or gently irrigate and flush the catheter with 0.9% sodium chloride solution. If these measures fail, suspect catheter clotting and notify the doctor, who may order instillation of a fibrinolytic or declotting agent.

Burning sensation. If the patient complains of burning around the port, the needle may have become dislodged, causing infiltration or extravasation. Edema may develop under the patient's arm or in the neck area. Stop the infusion and, if you suspect infiltration, notify the doctor.

Treatment usually requires reaccessing the port and verifying needle placement. If you suspect extravasation, don't remove the needle. Follow the facility's policy for treating extravasation, notify the doctor, and be prepared to administer the prescribed antidote.

"Twiddler's syndrome." If your patient repeatedly touches the port area, the VAP may rotate or the catheter may migrate. (Catheter migration also can occur for no apparent reason.) To correct such problems, loop and tape the catheter securely, apply a transparent semipermeable dressing, and advise the patient not to manipulate the device.

"Pinch-off syndrome." If the catheter becomes pinched between muscles in the patient's upper chest, you're able to infuse fluid but unable to get a blood return. More a nuisance than a complication, this syndrome requires surgical correction.

Other central venous insertion sites

An alternative to centrally inserted infusion sites, a peripherally inserted central catheter (PICC) rests in one of the vessels that directly enter the superior vena cava. PICC lines use the cephalic and basilic veins, which merge into the axillary vein and then the subclavian vein. The small diameters of these lines make them easier to insert and more comfortable for patients. PICC lines are preferable to central venous lines for patients with chest injury; chest, neck, or shoulder burns; or impaired respiratory function; when the patient's surgical site interferes with catheter placement, or when a doctor is unavailable to insert a central venous line. (See *Using a PICC.*)

Another alternative is the midline catheter (MLC), which is placed between the antecubital area and the head of the clavicle. This catheter placement is appropriate for therapy lasting 1 to 8 weeks and avoids placement in the superior vena cava.

Both MLC lines and PICC lines are being used more frequently in home care.

Using a PICC

A peripherally inserted central catheter (PICC), which has a smaller diameter, may be easier to insert than other central venous devices and provides safe, reliable access for chemotherapeutic and other drugs and blood sampling. Increasingly, PICC lines are used in home care. The patient receiving PICC therapy must have a peripheral vein large enough to accept a 14G or 16G introducer needle and a 3.8G to 4.8G catheter. The doctor or nurse inserts a PICC via the basilic, median antecubital basilic, cubital, or cephalic vein and then threads it to the superior vena cava or subclavian vein or to a noncentral site, such as the axillary vein.

Administration guidelines

Before infusing a chemotherapeutic drug through a PICC line, check for a blood return and flush the line with 0.9% sodium chloride solution. First, clamp the 7" (17.8-cm) extension tubing and connect the empty syringe to the tubing. Release the clamp, and aspirate slowly to verify blood return. Flush with 3 ml of the sodium chloride solution. Then administer the drug.

Afterward, flush again with 3 ml of the 0.9% sodium chloride solution. (Remember to flush with the same solution between infusions of incompatible drugs or fluids.)

Changing the dressing

Change the dressing every 4 days for an inpatient and every 5 to 7 days for a home care patient. If possible, choose a transparent semipermeable dressing, which has a high moisture-vapor transmission rate. Always use aseptic technique.

Complications

PICC therapy causes fewer and less severe complications than conventional central venous lines.

Phlebitis, perhaps the most common complication, may occur during the first 48 to 72 hours after PICC insertion. It's more common in left-sided or with large-gauge needle insertions. If phlebitis develops, apply warm, wet compresses to the upper arm, elevate the area, and encourage mild exercise. If phlebitis persists or worsens, remove the catheter, as ordered.

Air embolism is less likely to occur with PICC therapy than with traditional central venous lines because a PICC is inserted below heart level.

Some patients complain of pain at the catheter insertion site, usually resulting from the chemical properties of the infused drug or fluid. Slowing the infusion rate and applying warm compresses should relieve such pain. Migration of the catheter tip may occur with vigorous flushing. Patients receiving chemotherapy are especially vulnerable to this complication because of changes in intrathoracic pressure that are associated with frequent nausea and vomiting. If the catheter fails to show a blood return, arrange for a chest X-ray to determine the position of the catheter tip.

(continued)

Catheter occlusion, a relatively common complication, may require declotting with administration of a fibrinolytic, such as urokinase. As ordered, give urokinase according to the manufacturer's recommendations to restore catheter patency.

ADVERSE REACTIONS

Chemotherapeutic drugs may cause adverse reactions, including bone marrow suppression leading to leukopenia, thrombocytopenia, or anemia; GI reactions, such as nausea and vomiting or stomatitis; and alopecia.

Bone marrow suppression

The most common and potentially most serious adverse reaction to chemotherapy, bone marrow suppression is indicated by leukopenia with granulocytopenia, thrombocytopenia, and anemia. Check for this reaction by monitoring the blood count nadir, which indicates when the patient is at greatest risk.

Although biological response modifiers have been used to accelerate blood cell recovery, you must teach the patient specific guidelines based on the hematologic factor effected. (For more information, see Chapter 6, "Biological Response Modifiers.") See the specific patient-teaching guidelines below.

Leukopenia and granulocytopenia

This reaction places the patient at increased risk for infection, especially if the granulocyte count drops below 1,000/mm³. Signs and symptoms include sore throat, fever, and malaise. Follow these patient-teaching guidelines to help prevent this reaction:
• Provide information about good hygiene, and assess the patient frequently for signs and symptoms of infection.
• Teach the patient to recognize and report the signs and symptoms of infection: fever, cough, sore throat, or a burning sensation on urination.

- Teach the patient how to take his own temperature, and advise the patient and caregiver to notify the physician if his temperature is above 101° F (38.3° C).
- Warn the patient to avoid crowds and exposure to persons with colds or the flu during the nadir.
- Warn the patient that the inflammatory response may be decreased and the complications of leukopenia more difficult to detect when the patient is receiving a corticosteroid.

Thrombocytopenia

Although it may accompany leukopenia, thrombocytopenia is probably more dangerous because the patient risks hemorrhage, particularly when the platelet count drops below 50,000/mm³. If the count drops below 20,000/mm³, the patient may require transfusion of platelets. Early signs of thrombocytopenia include bleeding gums, increased bruising or petechiae, hypermenorrhea, tarry stools, hematuria, and coffee-ground vomitus. Use these teaching guidelines for the patient with the potential for thrombocytopenia:

- Advise the patient to avoid cuts and bruises and to use a soft toothbrush and an electric razor.
- Tell the patient to report sudden headaches, which could indicate potentially fatal intracranial bleeding.
- Instruct the patient to use a stool softener, as prescribed, to prevent colonic irritation and bleeding.
- Tell the patient not to use a rectal thermometer.
- Advise the patient that I.M. or S.C. injections should be avoided. If he is currently receiving medications by those routes, he should notify his doctor.

Anemia

This reaction may develop slowly over several courses of treatment. Signs and symptoms of anemia include, dizziness, fatigue, pallor, and shortness of breath after minimal exertion.

You will need to monitor the patient's hematocrit and hemoglobin levels and RBC counts. *Note:* The patient who is dehydrated from nausea, vomiting, or anorexia may exhibit a false-normal hematocrit level. Be prepared to administer a blood transfusion to a symptomatic patient. Follow these patient-teaching guidelines to help prevent anemia.

- Advise the patient to rest more frequently.
- Suggest that the patient increase dietary intake of iron-rich foods and take a multivitamin with iron, as prescribed.

GI reactions

The GI tract is extremely vulnerable to the cytotoxic effects of chemotherapy because the cells of the GI epithelium proliferate rapidly. The most common distressing GI effects for patients are nausea and vomiting. Patients may also develop stomatitis.

Nausea and vomiting

Gastric mucosal irritation, chemical irritation of the central nervous system, or psychogenic factors may cause this reaction. Managing these symptoms may require an antiemetic or combination therapy. For more specific guidelines, see Chapter 9, "Pharmacologic Management of Adverse Reactions."

Stomatitis

Stomatitis, which is a temporary reaction, can range from mild and barely noticeable to severe and debilitating. Symptoms may appear as soon as 3 days after beginning chemotherapy and include increased sensitivity to hot and cold liquids, intolerance to fruit juices, and redness of the oral mucosa. For guidelines to help the patient prevent and deal with this reaction, also see Chapter 9.

Alopecia

Although alopecia is not treatable, good patient teaching can help the patient deal with this distressing adverse reaction. Follow the guidelines listed below:

- Prepare the patient for alopecia, informing him that hair loss typically occurs gradually and reverses after treatment ends.
- Tell the patient that alopecia may be partial or complete, that it affects both men and women, and that it may affect the scalp, eyebrows, eyelashes, and body hair.

POINTS TO REMEMBER

Administering chemotherapy is a skill that requires extensive knowledge and careful consideration. The patient receiving chemotherapeutic drugs needs reassurance and information, and those who handle and administer such drugs must do so with care.

Remember these guidelines when providing care for the patient receiving chemotherapeutic drugs:

- Understand the risks of handling chemotherapeutic drugs, and take precautions to properly prepare, administer, and dispose of such drugs according to the manufacturer's instructions and your facility's policy. Become familiar with safety equipment and use it whenever handling chemotherapeutic drugs.
- Learn the various methods of administering chemotherapy, including central venous administration, VAP placement, and placement of PICC lines. Remember always to wear gloves and use aseptic technique when inserting and removing I.V. lines.
- Be alert for signs of complications and adverse reactions, and understand how to treat and prevent them.
- Provide the patient and family with information on identifying adverse reactions and properly disposing of chemotherapeutic drugs and bodily fluids.

When administered with care, chemotherapeutic drugs can effectively contribute to cancer treatment. When you understand the nuances of chemotherapy, you can protect yourself and provide the best patient care.

Alkylating agents

busulfan	ifosfamide
carboplatin	lomustine
carmustine	mechlorethamine hydrochloride
chlorambucil	melphalan
cisplatin	pipobroman
cyclophosphamide	thiotepa
dacarbazine	uracil mustard

Alkylating agents are cell-cycle nonspecific. Varying degrees of specificity exist among the different agents. They are polyfunctional compounds that can be divided chemically into five groups: nitrogen mustards, ethylenimines, alkylsulfonates, triazenes, and nitrosoureas. They are often effective against tumors with large volumes and slow cell turnover rate.

Pharmacology

Alkylating agents are highly reactive, primarily targeting nucleic acids and forming covalent linkages with the nucleophilic centers in many different kinds of molecules. Their polyfunctional character allows them to cross-link double-stranded DNA, preventing the strands from separating for replication, which appears to contribute more to the cytotoxic effects of these agents than other results of alkylation.

Clinical indications and actions

Alkylating agents are useful alone or in combination with other types of antineoplastic agents for the treatment of a variety of tumors. See the individual agents for specific uses.

Overview of adverse reactions

The most frequent adverse reactions to alkylating agents include bone marrow depression, leukopenia, thrombocytopenia, fever, chills, sore throat, nausea, vomiting, diarrhea, flank or joint pain, anxiety, swelling of feet or lower legs, hair loss, and redness or pain at injection site.

Special considerations

- Follow all established procedures for safe and proper handling, administration, and disposal of chemotherapeutic drugs.
- Vital signs and patency of catheter or I.V. line should be monitored throughout administration.
- Treat extravasation promptly.
- Attempt to alleviate or reduce anxiety in patient and family before treatment.
- Monitor BUN, hematocrit level, platelet count, ALT (formerly SGPT), AST (formerly SGOT), LDH, serum bilirubin, serum creatinine, uric acid, total and differential WBC counts, and other levels as required for the specific agent.

Information for the patient

- Tell patient to avoid exposure to persons with bacterial or viral infections because chemotherapy can increase susceptibility to infection. Patient should report any signs of infection promptly.
- Instruct patient in proper oral hygiene, including caution when using toothbrush, dental floss, and toothpicks.

- Tell patient to complete dental work before therapy begins, whenever possible, or to delay it until blood counts are normal.
- Warn patient that he may bruise easily because of drug's effect on blood counts.

busulfan
Myleran
Pregnancy risk category: D

How supplied

Tablets (scored): 2 mg

Indications, route, and dosage

Indications and dosage may vary. Check current literature for recommended protocol.
Chronic myelogenous leukemia (CML)
Adults: 4 to 8 mg P.O. daily, but may range from 1 to 12 mg P.O. daily (0.06 mg/kg or 1.8 mg/m²).
Children: 0.06 to 0.12 mg/kg or 1.8 to 4.6 mg/m² P.O. daily.

Pharmacodynamics

Busulfan is an alkylating agent that exerts its cytotoxic activity by interfering with DNA replication and RNA transcription, causing a disruption of nucleic acid function.

Pharmacokinetics

Absorption: Busulfan is well absorbed from the GI tract.
Distribution: Distribution into the brain and CSF is unknown.
Metabolism: Busulfan is metabolized in the liver.
Excretion: Busulfan is cleared rapidly from the plasma. Busulfan and its metabolites are excreted in urine.

Contraindications and precautions

Busulfan is contraindicated in patients with a history of resistance to previous therapy with the drug.
    Busulfan should be used with caution in men and women of childbearing age because it can impair fertility, in

---

those with a history of gout because of its hyperuricemic effects, and in patients whose immune system is compromised because of the potential for additive toxicity. The drug can cause further myelosuppression, increasing the patient's risk of infection.

Interactions

None reported.

Effects on diagnostic tests

Drug-induced cellular dysplasia may interfere with interpretation of cytologic studies.

Busulfan therapy may increase blood and urine levels of uric acid as a result of the increased purine catabolism that accompanies cell destruction.

Adverse reactions

DERM: transient hyperpigmentation, anhidrosis.
GI: nausea, vomiting, diarrhea, cheilosis, glossitis, stomatitis.
GU: amenorrhea, testicular atrophy, renal calculi, uric acid nephropathy, impotence.
HEMA: *bone marrow depression* (dose-limiting); WBC count falling after about 10 days and continuing to fall for 2 weeks after stopping drug; *thrombocytopenia, leukopenia,* anemia.
Hepatic: cholestatic jaundice.
Metabolic: Addison-like wasting syndrome, profound hyperuricemia from increased cell lysis.
Other: gynecomastia, alopecia, *irreversible pulmonary fibrosis (commonly termed "busulfan lung")*, cellular dysplasia.

Note: Consider discontinuing the drug if the WBC count decreases to approximately 15,000/mm^3, or if patient's clinical symptoms and changes on chest X-ray support a finding of pulmonary fibrosis.

Overdose and treatment

Clinical manifestations of overdose include hematologic changes such as leukopenia and thrombocytopenia.

Treatment is supportive and includes transfusion of blood components and antibiotics for any infections that develop.

Special considerations

- Busulfan is less effective in patients with CML who lack the Philadelphia (Ph^1) chromosome. Drug is also not effective in treating chronic lymphocytic leukemia, acute leukemia, or the blastic crisis of CML.
- Avoid all I.M. injections when the platelet count is below 100,000/mm^3.
- Patient response (increased appetite, sense of well-being, decreased total WBC count, reduction in size of spleen) usually begins 1 to 2 weeks after initiating the drug.
- Use cautiously in patients recently given other myelosuppressive drugs or radiation treatment and in those with depressed neutrophil or platelet count.
- Watch for signs of infection (fever, sore throat).
- Pulmonary fibrosis may be delayed for 4 to 6 months.
- Persistent cough and progressive dyspnea with alveolar exudate may result from drug toxicity, not pneumonia. Instruct patient to report symptoms so that dose can be adjusted.
- Monitor uric acid levels, CBC, and kidney function.

Information for the patient

- Recommend that patient take contraceptive measures during therapy.
- Advise patient to use aspirin-containing products cautiously and to watch closely for signs of bleeding and report them promptly.
- Tell patient to take medication at the same time each day.
- Emphasize the importance of continuing to take medication despite nausea and vomiting.
- Advise patient to take the drug on an empty stomach if nausea is a problem.
- Instruct patient about the signs and symptoms of infection, and tell him to report them promptly.

carboplatin
Paraplatin
Pregnancy risk category: D

How supplied

Injection: 50-mg, 150-mg, 450-mg vials

Indications, route, and dosage

Palliative treatment of ovarian cancer
Women: Initial recommended dose is 360 mg/m^2 I.V. on day 1. Dose is repeated q 4 weeks. Dosage adjustments are based on the lowest posttreatment platelet or neutrophil value obtained in weekly blood counts.

Lowest platelet count (per mm^3)	Lowest neutrophil count (per mm^3)	Adjusted dose
> 100,000	> 2,000	125%
50,000 to 100,000	500 to 2,000	No adjustment
< 50,000	< 500	75%

Pharmacodynamics

Carboplatin, a platinum coordination compound, causes cross-linking of DNA strands. Like cisplatin, carboplatin produces intrastrand and interstrand DNA cross-links rather than protein DNA cross-links.

Pharmacokinetics

Absorption: Carboplatin is administered I.V.
Distribution: Carboplatin's volume of distribution is approximately equal to total body water; no significant protein binding occurs.
Metabolism: Carboplatin is hydrolyzed to form hydroxylated and aquated species.
Excretion: 65% of the drug is excreted by the kidneys within 12 hours, 71% within 24 hours. Free platinum exhibits a half-life of 5 hours. Enterohepatic recirculation may occur.

Contraindications and precautions

Carboplatin is contraindicated in patients with a history of hypersensitivity to cisplatin, platinum-containing compounds, or mannitol. Avoid use in patients with severe bone marrow depression or bleeding. Transfusions may be necessary during treatment due to cumulative anemia. Bone marrow depression may be more severe in patients with creatinine clearance less than 60 ml/minute. Patients over age 65 are at greater risk for neurotoxicity.

Use with caution in patients with decreased renal function; use adjusted dose. Exercise extreme caution when preparing or administering carboplatin to avoid mutagenic, teratogenic, and carcinogenic risks. Use a biological safety cabinet, wear gloves and mask, and use syringes with luerlock fittings to prevent leakage of drug solution. Also correctly dispose of needles, vials, and unused drug, and avoid contaminating work surfaces. Avoid inhalation of dust or vapors and contact with skin or mucous membranes.

Interactions

Concomitant use with nephrotoxic agents produces additive nephrotoxicity. Concomitant use with phenytoin may decrease phenytoin serum levels.

Effects on diagnostic tests

High doses of carboplatin may cause elevated bilirubin, alkaline phosphatase, AST (formerly SGOT), serum creatinine, and blood urea levels.

Adverse reactions

CNS: peripheral neuropathy.
GI: constipation, diarrhea, nausea, vomiting, electrolyte loss.
HEMA: *bone marrow depression, thrombocytopenia, leukopenia,* neutropenia, anemia.
Hepatic: hepatotoxicity, pain.
Local: pain at injection site.
Other: alopecia, *hypersensitivity,* ototoxicity, pain, asthenia.

Overdose and treatment

Symptoms of overdose result from bone marrow suppression or hepatotoxicity. There is no known antidote for carboplatin overdose.

Special considerations

Besides those relevant to all alkylating agents, consider the following recommendations.
- Reconstitute with dextrose 5% in water (D_5W), 0.9% sodium chloride solution, or sterile water for injection to make a concentration of 10 mg/ml.
- Carboplatin can be diluted with 0.9% sodium chloride solution or D_5W.
- Unopened vials should be stored at room temperature. Once reconstituted and diluted as directed, solution is stable at room temperature for 8 hours. Because the drug does not contain antibacterial preservatives, unused drug should be discarded after 8 hours.
- Do not use needles or I.V. administration sets containing aluminum because carboplatin may precipitate and lose potency.
- Although carboplatin is promoted as causing less nausea and vomiting than cisplatin, it can cause severe emesis. Administer antiemetic therapy.
- Administration of carboplatin requires the supervision of a doctor experienced in the use of chemotherapeutic drugs.

Information for the patient
- Stress importance of adequate fluid intake and increase in urine output to facilitate uric acid excretion.
- Tell patient to report tinnitus immediately to prevent permanent hearing loss. Patient should have audiometric test before initial course of therapy and before subsequent courses.
- Advise patient to avoid exposure to persons with infections.
- Tell patient to promptly report any unusual bleeding or bruising.

Geriatric use
Patients over age 65 are at greater risk for neurotoxicity.

---

carmustine (BCNU)
BiCNU
Pregnancy risk category: D

How supplied

Injection: 100-mg vial (lyophilized), with a 3-ml vial of absolute alcohol supplied as a diluent

Indications, route, and dosage

Indications and dosage may vary. Check current literature for recommended protocol.
Brain, colon, and stomach cancers; Hodgkin's disease; non-Hodgkin's lymphomas; melanomas; multiple myeloma; hepatoma
Adults: 75 to 100 mg/m^2 by slow I.V. infusion daily for 2 consecutive days, repeated q 6 weeks if platelet count is above 100,000/mm^3 and WBC count is above 4,000/mm^3. Reduce dosage by 50% when WBC count is below 2,000/mm^3 and platelet count is below 25,000/mm^3.
Alternate therapy: 200 mg/m^2 by slow I.V. infusion as a single dose, repeated q 6 to 8 weeks; or 40 mg/m^2 by slow I.V. infusion for 5 consecutive days, repeated q 6 weeks.

Pharmacodynamics

The cytotoxic action of carmustine is mediated through its metabolites, which inhibit several enzymes involved with DNA formation. This agent can also cause cross-linking of DNA. Cross-linking interferes with DNA, RNA, and protein synthesis. Cross-resistance between carmustine and lomustine has been known to occur.

Pharmacokinetics

Absorption: Carmustine must be administered I.V. and is not absorbed across the GI tract.
Distribution: Carmustine is cleared rapidly from the plasma. After I.V. administration, carmustine and its metabolites distribute rapidly into the CSF. Carmustine also is distributed in breast milk.
Metabolism: Carmustine is metabolized in the liver.

Excretion: Approximately 60% to 70% of carmustine and its metabolites are excreted in urine within 96 hours, 6% to 10% is excreted as carbon dioxide by the lungs, and 1% is excreted in feces. Enterohepatic circulation and storage of the drug in adipose tissue can occur and may cause delayed hematologic toxicity.

Contraindications and precautions

Carmustine is contraindicated in patients with a history of hypersensitivity to the drug.

Drug should be withheld or dosage reduced in the presence of hepatic or renal insufficiency because drug accumulation may occur; in patients with compromised hematologic status because of the drug's adverse hematologic effects; and in patients with recent exposure to cytotoxic medications or radiation therapy.

Interactions

Concomitant use with cimetidine increases the bone marrow toxicity of carmustine. The mechanism of this interaction is unknown. Avoid concomitant use of these drugs.

Effects on diagnostic tests

Carmustine therapy may increase BUN, serum alkaline phosphatase, AST (formerly SGOT), and bilirubin concentrations.

Adverse reactions

DERM: hyperpigmentation on accidental contact of drug with skin; alopecia.
GI: nausea, possibly severe, lasting 2 to 6 hours after dose; vomiting.
GU: nephrotoxicity.
HEMA: *bone marrow depression* (dose-limiting and usually occurring 4 to 6 weeks after a dose), *leukopenia, thrombocytopenia,* anemia.
Hepatic: hepatotoxicity.
Metabolic: possible hyperuricemia in lymphoma patients when rapid cell lysis occurs.
Local: intense pain at infusion site.

Other: *pulmonary fibrosis.*

Overdose and treatment

Clinical manifestations of overdose include leukopenia, thrombocytopenia, nausea, and vomiting.

Treatment consists of supportive measures, including transfusion of blood components, administration of antibiotics for any infections that develop, and administration of antiemetics.

Special considerations

- Reconstitute the 100-mg vial with the 3 ml of absolute alcohol provided by the manufacturer, then dilute further with 27 ml sterile water for injection. Resultant solution contains carmustine 3.3 mg/ml in 10% ethanol. Dilute in 0.9% sodium chloride solution or dextrose 5% in water for I.V. infusion. Give at least 250 ml over 1 to 2 hours. Discard excess drug.
- Wear gloves to administer carmustine infusion and when changing I.V. tubing. Avoid contact with skin because carmustine will cause a brown stain. If drug comes into contact with skin, wash off thoroughly.
- Solution is unstable in plastic I.V. bags. Administer only in glass containers.
- Carmustine may decompose at temperatures above 80° F (26.6° C).
- If powder liquefies or appears oily, it should be discarded; this is a sign of decomposition.
- Reconstituted solution may be stored in refrigerator for 24 hours.
- Don't mix with other drugs during administration.
- Avoid all I.M. injections when platelet count is below 100,000/mm^3.
- To reduce pain on infusion, dilute further or slow infusion rate.
- Intense flushing of the skin may occur during I.V. infusion, but usually disappears within 2 to 4 hours.
- To reduce nausea, give antiemetic before administering.
- Monitor CBC.
- Consider that pulmonary toxicity is more likely in people who smoke.

- At first sign of extravasation, infusion should be discontinued and area infiltrated with liberal injections of 0.5 mEq/ml sodium bicarbonate solution.
- Carmustine has been applied topically in concentrations of 0.5% to 2% to treat mycosis fungoides.
- Prescribe anticoagulants and aspirin products cautiously. Monitor patient closely for signs of bleeding.
- Because carmustine crosses the blood-brain barrier, it may be used to treat primary brain tumors.

Information for the patient
- Warn patient to watch for signs of infection (fever, sore throat) and bone marrow toxicity (anemia, fatigue, easy bruising, nose or gum bleeding, melena). Tell patient to take temperature daily.
- Remind patient to return for follow-up blood tests weekly, or as needed, and to watch for signs and symptoms of infection.
- Advise patient to avoid exposure to persons with infections.
- Tell patient to avoid nonprescription products containing aspirin because they may precipitate bleeding. Advise patient to report any signs of bleeding promptly.
- Advise patient not to smoke because of increased risk of pulmonary toxicity.

chlorambucil
Leukeran
Pregnancy risk category: D

How supplied

Tablets (sugar-coated): 2 mg

Indications, route, and dosage

Indications and dosage may vary. Check current literature for recommended protocol.

Chronic lymphocytic leukemia, diffuse lymphocytic lymphoma, Hodgkin's disease, autoimmune hemolytic anemias, lupus erythematosus, glomerulonephritis, nephrotic syndrome, polycythemia vera, macroglobulinemia, ovarian neoplasms
Adults: 100 to 200 mcg/kg or 3 to 6 mg/m² P.O. daily as a single dose or in divided doses for 3 to 6 weeks. Usual dose is 4 to 10 mg daily. Reduce dose if within 4 weeks of a full course of radiation therapy.
Children: 100 to 200 mcg/kg or 4.5 mg/m² P.O. as a single daily dose.

Pharmacodynamics

Chlorambucil exerts its cytotoxic activity by cross-linking strands of cellular DNA and RNA, disrupting normal nucleic acid function.

Pharmacokinetics

Absorption: Chlorambucil is well absorbed from the GI tract.
Distribution: The distribution of chlorambucil is not well understood. However, the drug and its metabolites have been shown to be highly bound to plasma and tissue proteins.
Metabolism: Chlorambucil is metabolized in the liver. The primary metabolite, phenylacetic acid mustard, also possesses cytotoxic activity.
Excretion: The metabolites of chlorambucil are excreted in urine. The half-life of the parent compound is 2 hours; that of the phenylacetic acid metabolite, 2¹/₂ hours. Chlorambucil is probably not dialyzable.

Contraindications and precautions

Chlorambucil is contraindicated in patients with a history of hypersensitivity to the drug or of resistance to previous therapy with the drug. Cross-sensitivity, which manifests as a rash, may occur between chlorambucil and other alkylating agents.

Dosage adjustments must be considered in patients with hematologic impairment because of the drug's hematologic toxicity.

Chlorambucil should be used with caution in patients with a history of seizures, head trauma, or use of epileptogenic drugs. There is a small risk of chlorambucil-induced seizure.

Because of the potential for additive toxicity, patients should not receive a full dose of chlorambucil if a full course of radiation therapy or other myelosuppressive drugs were administered within the preceding 4 weeks.

Interactions

None reported.

Effects on diagnostic tests

Chlorambucil therapy may increase concentrations of serum alkaline phosphatase, AST (formerly SGOT), and blood and urine uric acid levels.

Adverse reactions

CNS: seizures (with high doses).
DERM: rash, pruritus, peripheral neuropathy (rare).
GI: nausea, vomiting, anorexia, abdominal pain, diarrhea.
GU: sterile cystitis (rare).
HEMA: *pancytopenia* (dose-limiting).
Metabolic: hyperuricemia.
Other: *pulmonary fibrosis*, drug fever, alopecia (rare).

Overdose and treatment

Clinical manifestations of overdose include reversible pancytopenia in adults and vomiting, ataxia, abdominal pain, muscle twitching, and major motor seizures in children.

Treatment is usually supportive, with transfusion of blood components if necessary and appropriate anticonvulsant therapy if seizures occur. Induction of emesis, activated charcoal, and gastric lavage may be useful in removing unabsorbed drug.

Special considerations

Besides those relevant to all alkylating agents, consider the following recommendations.
• Oral suspension can be prepared in the pharmacy by crushing tablets and mixing powder with a suspending agent and simple syrup.

- Avoid all I.M. injections when platelet count is below 100,000/mm^3.
- Anticoagulants and aspirin products should be used cautiously. Watch closely for signs of bleeding.
- Chlorambucil-induced pancytopenia generally lasts 1 to 2 weeks but may persist for 3 to 4 weeks. It is reversible up to a cumulative dose of 6.5 mg/kg in a single course.
- To prevent hyperuricemia with resulting uric acid nephropathy, allopurinol may be used with adequate hydration. Monitor uric acid.
- Store tablets in a tightly closed, light-resistant container.

Information for the patient
- Emphasize importance of continuing medication despite nausea and vomiting, and of keeping appointments for periodic blood work.
- Advise patient to call if vomiting occurs shortly after taking the dose or if symptoms of infection or bleeding are present.
- Tell patient to avoid exposure to persons with infections.
- Instruct patient to avoid nonprescription products containing aspirin.

cisplatin (cis-platinum)
Platinol, Platinol AQ

Pregnancy risk category: D

How supplied
Injection: 10-mg, 50-mg vials (lyophilized); 50-mg, 100-mg vials (aqueous)

Indications, route, and dosage
Indications and dosage may vary. Check current literature for recommended protocol.
Adjunctive therapy in metastatic testicular cancer
Men: 20 mg/m^2 I.V. daily for 5 days. Repeat q 3 weeks for three cycles or more. Usually used in therapeutic regimen with bleomycin and vinblastine.

Adjunctive therapy in metastatic ovarian cancer; head and neck, lung, and esophageal cancers
Adults: 100 mg/m² I.V. repeated q 4 weeks, or 50 mg/m² I.V. q 3 weeks with concurrent doxorubicin hydrochloride therapy (ovarian cancer only). Give as I.V. infusion in 1 liter of solution with 37.5 g mannitol over 6 to 8 hours.

Treatment of advanced bladder cancer
Adults: 50 to 70 mg/m² I.V. q 3 to 4 weeks. Patients who have received other antineoplastic agents or radiation therapy should receive 50 mg/m² q 4 weeks.

Note: Prehydration and mannitol diuresis may reduce renal toxicity and ototoxicity significantly.

Pharmacodynamics

Cisplatin exerts its cytotoxic effects by binding with DNA and inhibiting DNA synthesis and, to a lesser extent, by inhibiting protein and RNA synthesis. Cisplatin also acts as a bifunctional alkylating agent, causing intrastrand and interstrand cross-links of DNA. Interstrand cross-linking appears to correlate well with the cytotoxicity of the drug.

Pharmacokinetics

Absorption: Cisplatin must be administered I.V.
Distribution: Cisplatin distributes widely into tissues, with the highest concentrations found in the kidneys, liver, and prostate gland. Cisplatin can accumulate in body tissues, with drug being detected up to 6 months after the last dose. Cisplatin does not readily cross the blood-brain barrier. The drug is extensively and irreversibly bound to plasma proteins and tissue proteins.
Metabolism: The metabolic fate of cisplatin is unclear.
Excretion: Cisplatin is excreted primarily unchanged in urine. In patients with normal renal function, the half-life of the initial elimination phase is about 25 to 79 minutes; the terminal phase half-life is about 58 to 78 hours. The terminal half-life of total platinum is up to 10 days.

Contraindications and precautions

Cisplatin is contraindicated in patients with a history of hypersensitivity to cisplatin or other platinum-containing compounds. Patients who have been previously exposed to these agents should undergo skin testing before cisplatin therapy because of potential for allergic reaction. The drug is also contraindicated in patients with myelosuppression or hearing impairment because it may worsen these conditions.

Cisplatin should be used with caution in patients with impaired renal function because of the drug's nephrotoxic effects. Dosage may need to be adjusted. Cisplatin is usually not used in patients with a creatinine clearance below 50 ml/minute. Perform baseline audiometry before therapy begins. Cisplatin can impair fertility. Aspermia has been reported after cisplatin therapy.

Interactions

Concomitant use with aminoglycosides potentiates the cumulative nephrotoxicity caused by cisplatin; additive toxicity is the mechanism for this interaction. Therefore, aminoglycosides should not be used within 2 weeks of cisplatin therapy. Concomitant use with loop diuretics increases the risk of ototoxicity; closely monitor the patient's audiologic status. Concomitant use with phenytoin may decrease serum concentration of phenytoin.

Effects on diagnostic tests

Cisplatin therapy may increase BUN, serum creatinine, and serum uric acid levels. It may decrease creatinine clearance as well as serum calcium, magnesium, phosphate, and potassium levels, indicating nephrotoxicity.

Adverse reactions

CNS: peripheral neuritis, loss of taste, *seizures,* headache. *(Note:* Drug should be discontinued if signs of neurotoxicity appear.)
EENT: tinnitus, high-frequency hearing loss (may occur in both ears).
GI: nausea and vomiting, beginning 1 to 4 hours after dose and lasting 24 hours; diarrhea; metallic taste; stomatitis.
GU: more prolonged and severe renal toxicity with repeated courses of therapy (dose-limiting).
HEMA: mild myelosuppression in 25% to 30% of patients; *leukopenia; thrombocytopenia;* anemia; nadirs in circulating

---

platelets and leukocytes on days 18 to 23, with recovery by day 39.

Other: anaphylactoid reaction, hyperuricemia, hypomagnesemia.

Overdose and treatment

Clinical manifestations of overdose include leukopenia, thrombocytopenia, nausea, and vomiting.

Treatment is generally supportive and includes transfusion of blood components, administration of antibiotics for possible infections, and administration of antiemetics. Cisplatin can be removed by dialysis, but only within 3 hours after administration.

Special considerations

Besides those relevant to all alkylating agents, consider the following recommendations.

- Review hematologic status and creatinine clearance before therapy.
- Reconstitute 10-mg vial with 10 ml and 50-mg vial with 50 ml of sterile water for injection to yield a concentration of 1 mg/ml. The drug may be diluted further in a solution containing sodium chloride for I.V. infusion.
- Do not use aluminum needles for reconstitution or administration of cisplatin; a black precipitate may form. Use stainless steel needles.
- Drug is stable for 24 hours in sodium chloride solutions at room temperature. Do not refrigerate because precipitation may occur. Discard any solution containing precipitate.
- Infusions are most stable in chloride-containing solutions, such as dextrose 5% in water in 0.45%, 0.3%, or 0.225% sodium chloride solution.
- Mannitol may be given as a 12.5-g I.V. bolus before starting cisplatin infusion. Follow by infusion of mannitol at rate up to 10 g/hour, as necessary, to maintain urine output during cisplatin infusion and for 6 to 24 hours after infusion.
- I.V. sodium thiosulfate may be administered with cisplatin infusion to decrease risk of nephrotoxicity.

- Hydrate the patient with 0.9% sodium chloride solution before giving drug. Maintain urine output of 100 ml/hour for 4 consecutive hours before and 24 hours after infusion.
- Hydrate patient by encouraging oral fluid intake when possible.
- Avoid all I.M. injections when platelet count is low.
- Nausea and vomiting may be severe and protracted (up to 24 hours). Monitor fluid intake and output. Continue I.V. hydration until patient can tolerate adequate oral intake. High-dose metoclopramide (2 mg/kg I.V.), sometimes with dexamethasone 10 to 20 mg I.V., has been used to prevent and treat nausea and vomiting. Many patients respond favorably to treatment with ondansetron. Pretreatment with this serotonin receptor antagonist should begin 30 minutes before cisplatin therapy.
- Treat extravasation with local injections of a $^1/_6$ M sodium thiosulfate solution (prepared by mixing 4 ml of sodium thiosulfate 10% and 6 ml of sterile water for injection).
- Monitor CBC, platelet count, and renal function studies before initial and subsequent doses. Do not repeat dose unless platelet count is over 100,000/mm^3, WBC count is over 4,000/mm^3, serum creatinine level is under 1.5 mg/dl, and BUN level is under 25 mg/dl.
- Renal toxicity becomes more severe with repeated doses. Renal function must return to normal before next dose can be given.
- Monitor electrolytes extensively; aggressive supplementation is often required after a course of therapy.
- Anaphylactoid reaction usually responds to immediate treatment with epinephrine, corticosteroids, or antihistamines.
- Drug is given with bleomycin and vinblastine for testicular cancer and with doxorubicin for ovarian cancer.
- Avoid contact with skin. If contact occurs, wash drug off immediately with soap and water.

Information for the patient
- Stress importance of adequate fluid intake and increase in urine output to facilitate uric acid excretion.
- Tell patient to report tinnitus immediately, to prevent permanent hearing loss. Patient should have audiometric tests

---

before initial course of cisplatin therapy and before subsequent courses.
- Advise patient to avoid exposure to persons with infections.
- Tell patient to promptly report any unusual bleeding or
bruising.

cyclophosphamide
Cytoxan, Neosar

Pregnancy risk category: D

How supplied

Tablets: 25 mg, 50 mg
Injection: 100-mg, 200-mg, 500-mg, 1-g, 2-g vials

Indications, route, and dosage

Indications and dosage may vary. Check literature for recommended protocol.
**Breast, head, neck, lung, and ovarian cancers; Hodgkin's disease;
chronic lymphocytic or myelocytic and acute lymphoblastic leukemia;
neuroblastoma; retinoblastoma; non-Hodgkin's lymphomas; multiple
myeloma; mycosis fungoides; sarcomas; severe rheumatoid disorders;
glomerular and nephrotic syndrome (in children); immunosuppression
after transplantation**
Adults: 40 to 50 mg/kg P.O. or I.V. in single dose or in two to
five doses, then adjust for maintenance; or 2 to 4 mg/kg P.O.
daily for 10 days, then adjust for maintenance. Maintenance
dosage, 1 to 5 mg/kg P.O. daily; 10 to 15 mg/kg I.V. q 7 to 10
days; or 3 to 5 mg/kg I.V. twice weekly.
Children: 2 to 8 mg/kg or 60 to 250 mg/m^2 P.O. or I.V. daily for
6 days (dosage depends on susceptibility of neoplasm);
divide oral dosages; give I.V. dosages once weekly. Maintenance dosage is 2 to 5 mg/kg or 50 to 150 mg/m^2 P.O. twice
weekly.
†Polymyositis
Adults: 1 to 2 mg/kg P.O. daily.
†Rheumatoid arthritis
Adults: 1.5 to 3 mg/kg P.O. daily.

---

*Canada only   †Off-label use   Italicized adverse reactions are life-threatening.

†**Wegener's granulomatosis**
Adults: 1 to 2 mg/kg P.O. daily (usually administered with prednisone).

Pharmacodynamics

The cytotoxic action of cyclophosphamide is mediated by its two active metabolites. These metabolites function as alkylating agents, preventing cell division by cross-linking DNA strands. This results in an imbalance of growth within the cell, leading to cell death. Cyclophosphamide also has significant immunosuppressive activity.

Pharmacokinetics

Absorption: Cyclophosphamide is almost completely absorbed from the GI tract at doses of 100 mg or less. Higher doses (300 mg) are approximately 75% absorbed.
Distribution: Cyclophosphamide is distributed throughout the body, although only minimal amounts have been found in saliva, sweat, and synovial fluid. The concentration in CSF is too low for treatment of meningeal leukemia. The active metabolites are approximately 50% bound to plasma proteins.
Metabolism: Cyclophosphamide is metabolized to its active form by hepatic microsomal enzymes. The activity of these metabolites is terminated by metabolism to inactive forms.
Excretion: Cyclophosphamide and its metabolites are eliminated primarily in urine, with 15% to 30% excreted as unchanged drug. The plasma half-life ranges from 4 to $6^1/_2$ hours.

Contraindications and precautions

Use cyclophosphamide with caution in young men and women of childbearing age because it may impair fertility; in pregnant patients because it may be fetotoxic; in lactating patients because of potential harm to the neonate; and in patients with myelosuppression or infections because of potentially severe immunosuppression.

Use cautiously in patients with severe leukopenia, thrombocytopenia, malignant cell infiltration of bone marrow, after recent radiation therapy or chemotherapy, and in hepatic or renal disease.

Interactions

Concomitant use of cyclophosphamide with barbiturates, phenytoin, or chloral hydrate increases the rate of metabolism of cyclophosphamide to toxic metabolites. These agents are known to be inducers of hepatic microsomal enzymes and should be discontinued before cyclophosphamide therapy begins.

Corticosteroids are known to initially inhibit the metabolism of cyclophosphamide, reducing its effect. Eventual reduction of dose or discontinuation of steroids may increase metabolism of cyclophosphamide to a toxic level. Other drugs that may inhibit cyclophosphamide metabolism include allopurinol, chloramphenicol, chloroquine, imipramine, phenothiazines, potassium iodide, and vitamin A.

Patients on cyclophosphamide therapy who receive succinylcholine as an adjunct to anesthesia may experience prolonged respiratory distress and apnea. This may occur up to several days after discontinuation of cyclophosphamide. The mechanism of this interaction is that cyclophosphamide depresses the activity of pseudocholinesterase, the enzyme responsible for the inactivation of succinylcholine. Use succinylcholine with caution or not at all.

Concomitant use of cyclophosphamide may potentiate the cardiotoxic effects of doxorubicin.

Effects on diagnostic tests

Cyclophosphamide may suppress positive reaction to *Candida*, mumps, tricophyton, and tuberculin skin tests. A false-positive result on the Papanicolaou test may occur. Cyclophosphamide therapy may also increase serum uric acid concentrations and decrease serum pseudocholinesterase concentrations.

Adverse reactions

CV: *cardiotoxicity* (with very high doses and in combination with doxorubicin), thrombophlebitis.
GI: anorexia; nausea and vomiting (beginning within 6 hours and lasting 4 hours); stomatitis; mucositis; diarrhea.
GU: gonadal suppression (may be irreversible), *hemorrhagic cystitis* (may develop in approximately 10% of patients because of poor hydration), bladder fibrosis, *nephrotoxicity*.

---

*Canada only   †Off-label use   Italicized adverse reactions are life-threatening.

(*Note:* Drug should be discontinued if hemorrhagic cystitis develops.)

HEMA: *bone marrow depression* (dose-limiting); *leukopenia* (nadir between days 8 and 15, recovery in 17 to 28 days); *thrombocytopenia;* anemia.

Metabolic: hyperuricemia, SIADH secretion (with high doses).

Other: reversible alopecia in 50% of patients, especially with high doses; secondary malignancies; *pulmonary fibrosis* (with high doses); fever; *anaphylaxis;* dermatitis.

Overdose and treatment

Clinical manifestations of overdose include myelosuppression, alopecia, nausea, vomiting, and anorexia.

Treatment is generally supportive and includes transfusion of blood components and administration of antiemetics. Cyclophosphamide is dialyzable.

Special considerations

Besides those relevant to all alkylating agents, consider the following recommendations.

- Follow the facility's guidelines for the safe preparation, administration, and disposal of chemotherapeutic drugs.
- Reconstitute vials with appropriate volume of bacteriostatic or sterile water for injection to give a concentration of 20 mg/ml.
- Reconstituted solution is stable 6 days if refrigerated or 24 hours at room temperature.
- Cyclophosphamide can be given by direct I.V. push into a running I.V. line or by infusion in 0.9% sodium chloride solution or dextrose 5% in water.
- Avoid all I.M. injections when platelet counts are low.
- Oral medication should be taken with or after a meal. Higher oral doses (400 mg) may be tolerated better if divided into smaller doses.
- Administration with cold foods such as ice cream may improve toleration of oral dose.
- Push fluids (3 liters daily) to prevent hemorrhagic cystitis. Some clinicians use uroprotectant agents such as mesna. Do not give cyclophosphamide at bedtime because infrequent voiding during the night puts the patient at risk for hemorrhagic cystitis. If cystitis occurs, discontinue the

drug. (Cystitis may develop months after therapy has been discontinued.)
- Reduce dosage of cyclophosphamide if patient is concomitantly receiving corticosteroid therapy and develops viral or bacterial infections.
- Monitor for cyclophosphamide toxicity if patient's corticosteroid therapy is discontinued.
- Monitor uric acid, CBC, and renal and hepatic functions.
- Observe for hematuria, and ask patient if he has pain on urination.
- Nausea and vomiting are most common with high doses of I.V. cyclophosphamide.
- The dosage of cyclophosphamide should be adjusted in patients with renal impairment.
- Cyclophosphamide has been used successfully to treat many nonmalignant conditions—for example, multiple sclerosis—because of its immunosuppressive activity.

Information for the patient
- Advise both male and female patients to practice contraception while taking this drug and for 4 months after; cyclophosphamide is potentially teratogenic.
- Tell woman who is breast-feeding to stop because drug is dangerous for the infant.
- Emphasize importance of continuing medication despite nausea and vomiting.
- Advise patient to report vomiting that occurs shortly after an oral dose.
- Warn patient that alopecia is likely to occur, but that it is reversible.
- Encourage adequate fluid intake to prevent hemorrhagic cystitis and to facilitate uric acid excretion.

dacarbazine
DTIC-Dome
Pregnancy risk category: C

How supplied
Injection: 100 mg, 200 mg

Indications, route, and dosage

Indications and dosage may vary. Check current literature for recommended protocol.

Metastatic malignant melanoma

Adults: 2 to 4.5 mg/kg or 70 to 160 mg/m^2 I.V. daily for 10 days, then repeat q 4 weeks as tolerated; or 250 mg/m^2 I.V. daily for 5 days, repeated at 3-week intervals.

Hodgkin's disease

Adults: 150 mg/m^2 I.V. for 5 days, repeated q 4 weeks; or 375 mg/m^2 on day 1, repeated q 15 days (usually used in combination with other antineoplastics).

Pharmacodynamics

Three mechanisms have been proposed to explain the cytotoxicity of dacarbazine: alkylation, in which DNA and RNA synthesis are inhibited; antimetabolite activity, as a false precursor for purine synthesis; and binding with protein sulfhydryl groups.

Pharmacokinetics

Absorption: Because of poor absorption from the GI tract, dacarbazine must be administered I.V.

Distribution: Dacarbazine is thought to localize in body tissues, especially the liver. The drug crosses the blood-brain barrier to a limited extent. It is minimally bound to plasma proteins.

Metabolism: Dacarbazine is rapidly metabolized in the liver to several compounds, some of which may be active.

Excretion: The elimination of dacarbazine occurs in a biphasic manner, with an initial phase half-life of about 19 minutes and a terminal phase half-life of about 5 hours in patients with normal renal and hepatic function. From 30% to 45% of a dose is excreted in urine.

Contraindications and precautions

Dacarbazine is contraindicated in patients with a history of hypersensitivity to the drug.

Interactions

None reported.

---

*Canada only   †Off-label use   Italicized adverse reactions are life-threatening.

Effects on diagnostic tests

Dacarbazine therapy causes transient increases in serum BUN, ALT (formerly SGPT), AST (formerly SGOT), and alkaline phosphatase levels.

Adverse reactions

CNS: confusion, headache, paresthesia.
DERM: phototoxicity, urticaria.
EENT: blurred vision.
GI: severe nausea and vomiting begin within 1 to 3 hours in 90% of patients, last 1 to 12 hours; anorexia.
HEMA: *bone marrow depression* (dose-limiting), *leukopenia and thrombocytopenia* (nadir between 3 and 4 weeks), anemia. (*Note:* Drug should be discontinued if hematopoietic toxicity is evident.)
Local: severe pain if I.V. infiltrates or if solution is too concentrated; tissue damage.
Other: flulike syndrome (fever, malaise, myalgia beginning 7 days after treatment is stopped and possibly lasting 7 to 21 days), alopecia, facial flushing.

Overdose and treatment

Clinical manifestations of overdose include myelosuppression and diarrhea.

Treatment is usually supportive and includes transfusion of blood components and monitoring of hematologic parameters.

Special considerations

Besides those relevant to all alkylating agents, consider the following recommendations.
- To reconstitute the drug for I.V. administration, use a volume of sterile water for injection that gives a concentration of 10 mg/ml (9.9 ml for 100-mg vial, 19.7 ml for 200-mg vial).
- Drug may be diluted further with dextrose 5% in water to a volume of 100 to 200 ml for I.V. infusion over 30 minutes. Increase volume or slow the rate of infusion to decrease pain at infusion site.
- Drug may be administered I.V. push over 1 to 2 minutes.

- A change in solution color from ivory to pink indicates some drug degradation. During infusion, protect the solution from light to avoid possible drug breakdown.
- Treat extravasation with application of hot packs; this may relieve burning sensation, local pain, and irritation.
- Discard refrigerated solution after 72 hours; room temperature solution, after 8 hours.
- Nausea and vomiting may be minimized by administering dacarbazine by I.V. infusion and by hydrating patient 4 to 6 hours before therapy.
- Monitor uric acid levels.
- Reduce dosage when giving repeated doses to a patient with severely impaired renal function.
- Use lower dose if renal function or bone marrow is impaired. Stop drug if WBC count falls to 3,000/mm^3 or platelet count drops to 100,000/mm^3. Monitor CBC.
- Monitor daily temperature. Observe for signs of infection.
- Avoid all I.M. injections when platelet count is below 100,000/mm^3.
- Anticoagulants and aspirin products should be used cautiously. Watch closely for signs of bleeding.

Information for the patient
- Advise patient to avoid sunlight and sunlamps for first 2 days after treatment.
- Tell patient to avoid contact with persons who have infections.
- Reassure patient that growth of hair should return after treatment has ended.
- Reassure patient that flulike syndrome may be treated with mild antipyretics such as acetaminophen.
- Tell patient to avoid aspirin and aspirin-containing products. Teach him the signs and symptoms of bleeding, and urge him to report them promptly.

ifosfamide
Ifex

Pregnancy risk category: C

How supplied

Injection: 1-g, 2-g, 3-g vials

Indications, route, and dosage

Indications and dosage may vary. Check current literature for recommended protocol.

Testicular cancer, †lung cancer, †Hodgkin's disease, †non-Hodgkin's lymphoma, †breast cancer, †acute and †chronic lymphocytic leukemia, †ovarian cancer, and †sarcomas

Adults and children: 700 to 1,000 mg/m^2/day I.V. for 5 days; 2,400 mg/m^2 I.V. daily for 3 days; or up to 5,000 mg/m^2 I.V. as a single dose. Regimen is usually repeated q 3 weeks.

Ifosfamide may be given by slow I.V. push, by intermittent infusion over at least 30 minutes, or by continuous infusion.

Pharmacodynamics

Ifosfamide requires activation by hepatic microsomal enzymes to exert its cytotoxic activity. The active compound cross-links strands of DNA and also breaks the DNA chain.

Pharmacokinetics

Absorption: Ifosfamide must be administered I.V.
Distribution: Ifosfamide crosses the blood-brain barrier, but its metabolites do not; therefore, alkylating activity does not occur in CSF.
Metabolism: Approximately 50% of a dose is metabolized in the liver.
Excretion: Ifosfamide and its metabolites are excreted primarily in the urine. The plasma elimination half-life is reported to be about 14 hours.

Contraindications and precautions

No contraindications are reported for ifosfamide. Dosage adjustments are necessary in patients with renal impairment.

---

*Canada only   †Off-label use   Italicized adverse reactions are life-threatening.

Interactions

Concomitant use with phenobarbital, phenytoin, and chloral hydrate may increase the activity of ifosfamide by induction of hepatic microsomal enzymes, increasing the conversion of ifosfamide to its active form. Concomitant corticosteroid therapy may decrease the effectiveness of ifosfamide by inhibiting the enzymes that convert the drug to its active form. Concurrent use of allopurinol may increase the activity and bone marrow toxicity of ifosfamide by prolonging its half-life by an unknown mechanism.

Effects on diagnostic tests

Ifosfamide therapy may increase serum concentrations of AST (formerly SGOT), ALT (formerly SGPT), bilirubin, LDH, creatinine, BUN, and alkaline phosphatase.

Adverse reactions

CNS: lethargy and confusion with high doses.
GI: nausea, vomiting.
GU: hemorrhagic cystitis (dose-limiting), nephrotoxicity, dysuria, urinary frequency.
HEMA: *leukopenia,* occasional thrombocytopenia.
Hepatic: elevated liver enzyme levels.
Other: alopecia, chemical phlebitis.

Overdose and treatment

Clinical manifestations of overdose include myelosuppression, nausea, vomiting, alopecia, and hemorrhagic cystitis.

Treatment is usually supportive and includes transfusion of blood components, administration of antiemetics, and bladder irrigation.

Special considerations

- Follow all established procedures for safe handling, administration, and disposal of chemotherapeutic drugs.
- To reconstitute 1-g vial, use 20 ml sterile water for injection to give a concentration of 50 mg/ml or 30 ml sterile water for injection to give a concentration of 100 mg/ml. A 0.9% sodium chloride solution may also be used for reconstitution.

---

*Canada only   †Off-label use   Italicized adverse reactions are life-threatening.

- Use reconstituted solution within 8 hours, because it contains no preservatives.
- Ifosfamide can be further diluted with dextrose 5% in water or 0.9% sodium chloride solution for I.V. infusion. This solution is stable for 7 days at room temperature.
- Ifosfamide may be given by I.V. push injection in a minimum of 75 ml of 0.9% sodium chloride solution over 30 minutes.
- I.V. infusions can be used to administer ifosfamide for up to 5 days.
- Push fluids (3 liters daily) and administer with mesna to prevent hemorrhagic cystitis. Avoid giving ifosfamide at bedtime, because infrequent voiding during the night may increase the possibility of cystitis. Bladder irrigation with 0.9% sodium chloride solution may decrease the likelihood of cystitis.
- Infusing each dose over 2 hours or longer will also decrease the possibility of cystitis.
- Sterile phlebitis may occur at the injection site; apply warm compresses.
- Encourage patient to void every 2 hours during the day and twice during the night. Catheterization may be required if patient is unable to void.
- Expect dosage adjustments in a patient with renal impairment. Closely monitor renal status throughout therapy.
- Assess patient for changes in mental status and cerebellar dysfunction. Dose may have to be decreased.
- Monitor CBC and renal and liver function tests.

Information for the patient
- Tell patient to ensure adequate fluid intake to prevent bladder toxicity and to facilitate uric acid excretion.
- Patient should avoid exposure to persons with infections.
- Reassure patient that hair should grow back after treatment has ended.
- Tell patient to call immediately if blood appears in the urine.

---

lomustine (CCNU)
CeeNU

Pregnancy risk category: C

How supplied

Capsules: 10 mg, 40 mg, 100 mg

Indications, route, and dosage

Indications and dosage may vary. Check current literature for recommended protocol.

Brain, colon, lung, and renal cell cancers; Hodgkin's disease; lymphomas; melanomas; multiple myeloma

Adults and children: 100 to 130 mg/m^2 P.O. as single dose q 6 weeks. Reduce dose according to bone marrow depression. Repeat doses should not be given until WBC count is greater than 4,000/mm^3 and platelet count is greater than 100,000/mm^3.

If WBC count is over 3,000/mm^3 and platelet count is over 75,000/mm^3, reduce subsequent doses by 25%; if WBC count is over 2,000/mm^3 and platelet count is over 50,000/mm^3, reduce subsequent doses by 50%; if WBC count is under 2,000/mm^3 and platelet count is under 25,000/mm^3, do not repeat dosage.

Pharmacodynamics

Lomustine exerts its cytotoxic activity through alkylation, resulting in the inhibition of DNA and RNA synthesis. As with other nitrosourea compounds, lomustine is known to modify cellular proteins and alkylate proteins, resulting in an inhibition of protein synthesis. Cross-resistance exists between lomustine and carmustine.

Pharmacokinetics

Absorption: Lomustine is rapidly and well absorbed across the GI tract after oral administration.
Distribution: Lomustine is distributed widely into body tissues. Because of its high lipid solubility, the drug and its metabolites cross the blood-brain barrier to a significant extent.

---

*Canada only   †Off-label use   Italicized adverse reactions are life-threatening.

Metabolism: Lomustine is metabolized rapidly and extensively in the liver. Some of the metabolites have cytotoxic activity.
Excretion: Metabolites of lomustine are excreted primarily in urine, with smaller amounts excreted in feces and through the lungs. The plasma elimination of lomustine is described as biphasic, with an initial phase half-life of 6 hours and a terminal phase of 1 to 2 days. The extended terminal phase half-life is thought to be caused by enterohepatic circulation and protein-binding.

Contraindications and precautions

Lomustine is contraindicated in patients with a history of hypersensitivity to the drug.

Lomustine should be used cautiously in patients with renal and hepatic dysfunction because drug accumulation may occur, and in patients with hematologic compromise and those who have recently received cytotoxic or radiation therapy because the drug's adverse hematologic effects may be exacerbated. Administer with caution to patients with infection because the drug is myelosuppressive and may exacerbate infections.

Interactions

None reported.

Effects on diagnostic tests

Lomustine therapy may cause transient increases in results of liver function tests.

Adverse reactions

CNS: lethargy, ataxia, dysarthria.
GI: nausea and vomiting, beginning within 4 to 5 hours and lasting 24 hours; stomatitis.
GU: nephrotoxicity, *progressive azotemia.*
HEMA: anemia, *bone marrow depression* (dose-limiting); *leukopenia,* delayed up to 6 weeks, lasting 1 to 2 weeks; *thrombocytopenia,* delayed up to 4 weeks, lasting 1 to 2 weeks.
Other: hepatotoxicity, alopecia.

Overdose and treatment

Clinical manifestations of overdose include myelosuppression, nausea, and vomiting.

Treatment is usually supportive and includes antiemetics and transfusion of blood components.

Special considerations

Besides those relevant to all alkylating agents, consider the following recommendations.

- Give 2 to 4 hours after meals. Lomustine will be more completely absorbed if taken when the stomach is empty. To prevent nausea, give antiemetic before administering.
- Anorexia may persist for 2 to 3 days after a given dose.
- Alcoholic beverages should be avoided for a short period after a dose of lomustine.
- Dose modification may be required in patients with decreased platelet, WBC, or RBC count.
- Monitor CBC weekly. Drug is usually not administered more often than every 6 weeks; bone marrow toxicity is cumulative and delayed.
- Frequently assess renal and hepatic status.
- Avoid all I.M. injections when platelet count is below 100,000/mm^3.
- Use anticoagulants cautiously. Watch closely for signs of bleeding.
- Because lomustine crosses the blood-brain barrier, it may be used to treat primary brain tumors.

Information for the patient

- Emphasize importance of continuing medication despite nausea and vomiting.
- Emphasize importance of taking the exact dose prescribed.
- Tell patient to call immediately if vomiting occurs shortly after a dose is taken.
- Advise patient to avoid exposure to persons with infections.
- Warn patient to avoid aspirin-containing products.
- Tell patient to promptly report a sore throat, fever, or any unusual bruising or bleeding.
- Tell woman who is breast-feeding to stop because of the risk to the infant.

mechlorethamine hydrochloride (nitrogen mustard)
Mustargen

Pregnancy risk category: D

How supplied

Injection: 10-mg vials
Topical solution: 10 mg in 5 to 10 ml 0.9% sodium chloride solution (must be prepared just before administration)
Ointment: 0.01% to 0.04%
    Must be compounded; not commercially available in the United States or Canada

Indications, route, and dosage

Indications and dosage may vary. Check current literature for recommended protocol.
Hodgkin's disease; non-Hodgkin's lymphomas; breast, lung, and ovarian cancer; diffuse lymphocytic lymphoma; multiple myeloma; chronic lymphocytic leukemia; mycosis fungoides; and polycythemia vera
Adults: 0.4 mg/kg I.V. as a single dose or 0.1 mg/kg I.V. on 4 successive days q 3 to 6 weeks. Give through running I.V. infusion. Dose reduced in prior radiation or chemotherapy to 0.2 to 0.4 mg/kg. Dose based on ideal or actual body weight, whichever is less.
Mycosis fungoides
Adults: Apply sufficient lotion or ointment to cover lesion one to four times a day for 6 to 12 months after a complete response. Continue maintenance treatments for up to 3 years.
Intracavitary doses for neoplastic effusions
Adults: 0.2 to 0.4 mg/kg.

Pharmacodynamics

Mechlorethamine exerts its cytotoxic activity through the basic processes of alkylation. The drug causes cross-linking of DNA strands, single-strand breakage of DNA, abnormal base pairing, and interruption of other intracellular processes, resulting in cell death.

---

*Canada only   †Off-label use   Italicized adverse reactions are life-threatening.

Pharmacokinetics

Absorption: Mechlorethamine is well absorbed after oral administration; however, because the drug is very irritating to tissue, it must be administered I.V. After intracavitary administration, mechlorethamine is absorbed incompletely, probably from deactivation by body fluids in the cavity.
Distribution: Mechlorethamine does not cross the blood-brain barrier.
Metabolism: Mechlorethamine is converted rapidly to its active form, which reacts quickly with various cellular components before being deactivated.
Excretion: Metabolites of mechlorethamine are excreted in urine. Less than 0.01% of an I.V. dose is excreted unchanged in urine.

Contraindications and precautions

Because of the potential of the drug to cause extensive and rapid development of amyloidosis, mechlorethamine is contraindicated in patients with foci of chronic or suppurative inflammation.

Use cautiously in the presence of severe anemia and depressed neutrophil or platelet count and in patients recently treated with radiation or chemotherapy.

It may be necessary to adjust dosage or discontinue therapy in patients with infections, hematologic compromise, or infiltration of the bone marrow by malignant cells because of the drug's adverse hematologic effects.

Interactions

None reported.

Effects on diagnostic tests

Mechlorethamine therapy may increase blood and urine uric acid levels and may decrease serum pseudocholinesterase concentrations.

Adverse reactions

CNS: drowsiness, vertigo, paresthesias (especially with high doses).

---

*Canada only   †Off-label use   Italicized adverse reactions are life-threatening.

EENT: tinnitus, metallic taste (immediately after dose), deafness.

GI: nausea, vomiting, and anorexia begin within 1 hour and last 8 to 24 hours.

GU: oligomenorrhea, amenorrhea, azoospermia, delayed spermatogenesis.

HEMA: *bone marrow depression* (dose-limiting) occurs by days 4 to 10, lasting 10 to 21 days; mild anemia begins in 2 to 3 weeks, possibly lasting 7 weeks.

Metabolic: hyperuricemia.

Local: thrombophlebitis, sloughing, severe irritation if drug extravasates or touches skin, rash.

Other: alopecia, herpes zoster.

Overdose and treatment

Clinical manifestations of overdose include lymphopenia and precipitation of uric acid crystals.

Treatment is usually supportive and includes transfusion of blood components, hydration, and allopurinol.

Special considerations

Besides those relevant to all alkylating agents, consider the following recommendations.

- To reconstitute powder, use 10 ml of sterile water for injection or 0.9% sodium chloride solution to give a concentration of 1 mg/ml.
- Solution is very unstable. It should be prepared immediately before infusion and used within 20 minutes. Discard unused solution.
- Drug may be administered by I.V. push over a few minutes into the tubing of a free-flowing I.V. infusion.
- Dilution of mechlorethamine into a large volume of I.V. solution is not recommended, because the drug may react with the diluent and is not stable for a prolonged period.
- Treatment of extravasation includes local injections of a $^1/_6$ M sodium thiosulfate solution. Prepare solution by mixing 4 ml of sodium thiosulfate 10% with 6 ml of sterile water for injection. Also apply ice packs for 6 to 12 hours to minimize local reactions.

- During intracavitary administration, patient should be turned from side to side every 15 minutes for 1 hour to distribute drug.
- Avoid contact with skin or mucous membranes. Wear gloves when preparing solution and during administration to prevent accidental skin contact. If contact occurs, wash with copious amounts of water.
- Monitor uric acid levels and CBC.
- To prevent hyperuricemia with resulting uric acid nephropathy, allopurinol may be given; keep patient well hydrated.
- Anticoagulants should be used cautiously. Watch closely for signs of bleeding.
- Avoid all I.M. injections when platelet count is low.

Information for the patient
- Tell patient to avoid exposure to persons with infections.
- Tell patient that adequate fluid intake is important to facilitate uric acid excretion.
- Reassure patient that hair should grow back after treatment has ended.
- Tell patient to promptly report any signs or symptoms of bleeding or infection.

melphalan (phenylalanine mustard)
Alkeran

Pregnancy risk category: D

How supplied

Tablets (scored): 2 mg

Indications, route, and dosage

Indications and dosage may vary. Check current literature for recommended protocol.
Multiple myeloma, testicular seminoma, non-Hodgkin's lymphoma, osteogenic sarcoma, breast cancer
Adults: 150 mcg/kg/day P.O. for 7 days, followed by a 3-week rest period. When WBC counts begin to rise, give maintenance dose of 50 mcg/kg. Alternatively, 100 to 500 mcg/kg/day P.O.

---

for 2 to 3 weeks or 250 mcg/kg/day for 4 days, followed by a 2- to 4-week rest period. When WBC counts begin to rise above 3,000/mm³ and platelet counts are greater than 100,000/mm³, give maintenance dose of 2 to 4 mg/day. Or 250 mcg/kg/day P.O. or 7 mg/m²/day P.O. for 5 days q 5 to 6 weeks. Adjust dose to maintain mild leukopenia and thrombocytopenia.

Nonresectable advanced ovarian cancer

Women: 200 mcg/kg/day P.O. for 5 days, repeated q 4 to 6 weeks if blood counts return to normal.

Pharmacodynamics

Melphalan exerts its cytotoxic activity by cross-linking strands of DNA and RNA and inhibiting protein synthesis.

Pharmacokinetics

Absorption: The absorption of melphalan from the GI tract is incomplete and variable. One study found that absorption ranged from 25% to 89% after an oral dose of 0.6 mg/kg.
Distribution: Melphalan distributes rapidly and widely into total body water. The drug initially is 50% to 60% bound to plasma proteins and eventually increases to 80% to 90% over time.
Metabolism: Melphalan is extensively deactivated by the process of hydrolysis.
Excretion: The elimination of melphalan has been described as biphasic, with an initial phase half-life of 8 minutes and a terminal half-life of 2 hours. Melphalan and its metabolites are excreted primarily in urine, with 10% of an oral dose excreted as unchanged drug.

Contraindications and precautions

Melphalan is contraindicated in patients with a history of hypersensitivity to the drug or resistance to previous therapy with it. Cross-sensitivity, which manifests as a rash, may occur between melphalan and chlorambucil.

Melphalan should be used with caution in patients with hematologic compromise or recent exposure to cytotoxic or radiation therapy because of the drug's myelosuppressive effects, and in patients with renal dysfunction because accumulation and excessive toxicity may occur.

Interactions

No significant drug interactions have been reported with melphalan.

Effects on diagnostic tests

Melphalan therapy may increase blood and urine levels of uric acid.

Adverse reactions

DERM: dermatitis.

GI: mild nausea and vomiting, diarrhea, stomatitis.

HEMA: *bone marrow depression* (dose-limiting); *leukopenia, thrombocytopenia, agranulocytosis;* acute nonlymphocytic leukemia may develop with chronic use. *(Note:* Drug should be discontinued at the first signs of bone marrow depression.)

Other: alopecia, pneumonitis, *pulmonary fibrosis.*

Overdose and treatment

Clinical manifestations of overdose include myelosuppression and hypocalcemia.

Treatment is usually supportive and includes transfusion of blood components.

Special considerations

Besides those relevant to all alkylating agents, consider the following recommendations.
- Oral dose may be taken all at one time.
- Administer melphalan on an empty stomach because absorption is decreased by food.
- Frequent hematologic monitoring, including CBC, is necessary for accurate dosage adjustments and prevention of toxicity.
- Discontinue therapy temporarily or reduce dosage if WBC count falls below 3,000/mm^3 or platelet count falls below 100,000/mm^3.
- Avoid I.M. injections when platelet count is below 100,000/mm^3.
- Anticoagulants, aspirin, and aspirin-containing products should be used cautiously.

---

*Canada only   †Off-label use   Italicized adverse reactions are life-threatening.

Information for the patient

- Tell patient it is vital to continue medication despite nausea and vomiting.
- Tell patient to call immediately if vomiting occurs shortly after taking a dose.
- Explain that adequate fluid intake is important to facilitate uric acid excretion.
- Advise patient to avoid exposure to persons with infections.
- Reassure patient that hair should grow back after treatment has ended.
- Tell patient to promptly report any signs and symptoms of infection or bleeding.

pipobroman
Vercyte

Pregnancy risk category: D

How supplied

Tablets: 25 mg

Indications, route, and dosage

Indications and dosage may vary. Check current literature for recommended protocol.

Polycythemia vera
Adults and children over age 15: 1 mg/kg P.O. daily for 30 days; may increase to 1.5 to 3 mg/kg P.O. daily until hematocrit level is reduced to 50% to 55%, then 0.1 to 0.2 mg/kg daily maintenance.

Chronic myelocytic leukemia
Adults and children over age 15: 1.5 to 2.5 mg/kg P.O. daily until WBC count drops to 10,000/mm^3; then start maintenance 7 mg to 175 mg daily. Stop drug if WBC count falls below 3,000/mm^3 or platelets fall below 150,000/mm^3.

Pharmacodynamics

Although pipobroman is classified as an alkylating agent, its exact mechanism of action is unknown.

Pharmacokinetics

Absorption: After oral administration, pipobroman is absorbed readily from the GI tract.
Distribution: Unknown.
Metabolism: Unknown.
Excretion: Unknown.

Contraindications and precautions

Pipobroman is contraindicated in patients with bone marrow depression resulting from radiation therapy or cytotoxic chemotherapy because of potential for additive bone marrow depression.

Interactions

Use cautiously in patients taking anticoagulants, and monitor for bleeding.

Effects on diagnostic tests

None reported.

Adverse reactions

DERM: rash.
GI: nausea, vomiting, abdominal cramps, diarrhea.
HEMA: *leukopenia, anemia, thrombocytopenia.*
   Note: Drug should be discontinued if adverse reactions persist.

Overdose and treatment

No information available.

Special considerations

• Administer in daily divided doses.
• Before therapy begins and periodically thereafter, perform liver and kidney function tests.
• Monitor CBC once or twice weekly and WBC counts every other day until desired result is obtained or toxic effects appear.
• Bone marrow studies should be performed before treatment begins and at time of maximal hematologic response. Bone marrow depression may not occur for 4

weeks or more after initiation of treatment. The WBC count is the most reliable index of bone marrow activity, but platelet count is also a helpful guide. Temporarily discontinue treatment if WBC count is below 3,000/mm³ or if platelet count is below 150,000/mm³. Treatment may be reinstated cautiously after blood counts rise.
• Dose-dependent anemia frequently develops. Dose reduction and blood transfusions usually reverse the anemia. Anemia caused by a hemolytic process is marked by a rapid drop in hemoglobin, increased bilirubin levels, and reticulocytosis. In this case, the drug should be discontinued.

Information for the patient
• Caution patient to call if nausea, vomiting, diarrhea, abdominal cramps, or skin rash become pronounced.
• Advise patient to use contraceptive measures during therapy.

thiotepa
Pregnancy risk category: D

How supplied
Injection: 15-mg vials

Indications, route, and dosage
Indications and dosage may vary. Check current literature for recommended protocol.
Breast, lung, and ovarian cancer; Hodgkin's disease; lymphomas
Adults and children age 12 and over: 0.2 mg/kg I.V. daily for 5 days, repeated q 2 to 4 weeks; or 0.3 to 0.4 mg/kg I.V. q 1 to 4 weeks.
Bladder tumor
Adults and children age 12 and over: 30 to 60 ml of a 1 mg/ml solution (thiotepa in distilled water) instilled in bladder once weekly for 4 weeks.
Neoplastic effusions
Adults and children age 12 and over: 0.6 to 0.8 mg/kg intracavitary or intratumor q 1 to 4 weeks.

Pharmacodynamics

Thiotepa exerts its cytotoxic activity as an alkylating agent, cross-linking strands of DNA and RNA and inhibiting protein synthesis, resulting in cell death.

Pharmacokinetics

Absorption: The absorption of thiotepa across the GI tract is incomplete. Absorption from the bladder is variable, ranging from 10% to 100% of an instilled dose. Absorption is increased by certain pathologic conditions. I.M. and pleural membrane absorption of thiotepa is also variable.
Distribution: Thiotepa crosses the blood-brain barrier.
Metabolism: Thiotepa is metabolized extensively in the liver.
Excretion: Thiotepa and its metabolites are excreted in urine.

Contraindications and precautions

Thiotepa is contraindicated in patients with a history of hypersensitivity to the drug and in patients with preexisting hepatic, renal, or bone marrow impairment, because of the potential for additive toxicity.

Interactions

When used concomitantly with succinylcholine, thiotepa may cause prolonged respirations and apnea. Thiotepa appears to inhibit the activity of pseudocholinesterase, the enzyme that deactivates succinylcholine. Use succinylcholine with extreme caution in patients receiving thiotepa.

Effects on diagnostic tests

Thiotepa therapy may increase blood and urine levels of uric acid and decrease plasma pseudocholinesterase concentrations.

Adverse reactions

CNS: dizziness.
DERM: hives, rash.
GI: nausea, vomiting, anorexia.
GU: amenorrhea, decreased spermatogenesis.
HEMA: *bone marrow depression* (dose-limiting), *leukopenia* (begins within 5 to 30 days), *thrombocytopenia, neutropenia,*

---

anemia. *(Note:* Drug should be discontinued if WBC or platelet count drops rapidly.)

Metabolic: hyperuricemia.

Local: intense pain at administration site.

Other: headache, fever, tightness of throat.

Overdose and treatment

Clinical manifestations of overdose include nausea, vomiting, and precipitation of uric acid in the renal tubules.

Treatment is usually supportive and includes transfusion of blood components, hydration, and administration of antiemetics and allopurinol.

Special considerations

- To reconstitute drug, use 1.5 ml of sterile water for injection to yield a concentration of 10 mg/ml. The solution is clear to slightly opaque.
- A 1 mg/ml solution is considered isotonic.
- Use only sterile water for injection to reconstitute. Refrigerated solution is stable for 5 days.
- Refrigerate dry powder; protect from light.
- Thiotepa can be given by all parenteral routes, including direct injection into the tumor.
- Stop drug or decrease dosage if WBC count falls below 4,000/mm^3 or if platelet count falls below 150,000/mm^3.
- Thiotepa may be mixed with procaine 2% or epinephrine 1:1,000, or both, for local use.
- Thiotepa may be further diluted to larger volumes with 0.9% sodium chloride solution, dextrose 5% in water, or lactated Ringer's solution for administration by I.V. infusion, intracavitary injection, or perfusion therapy.
- Withhold fluids for 8 to 10 hours before bladder instillation. Instill 60 ml of drug into bladder by catheter; ask patient to retain solution for 2 hours. Volume may be reduced to 30 ml if discomfort is too great. Reposition patient every 15 minutes for maximum area contact.
- To prevent hyperuricemia with resulting uric acid nephropathy, allopurinol may be given; keep patient well hydrated. Monitor uric acid.
- Monitor CBC weekly for at least 3 weeks after last dose. Warn patient to report even mild infections.

Canada only   †Off-label use   Italicized adverse reactions are life-threatening.

- Avoid all I.M. injections when platelet count is below 100,000/mm^3.
- Anticoagulants and aspirin products should be used cautiously. Watch closely for signs of bleeding. Instruct patient to avoid nonprescription products containing aspirin.
- Toxicity may be delayed and prolonged because drug binds to tissues and stays in body several hours.
- GU adverse reactions are reversible in 6 to 8 months.

Information for the patient
- Encourage patient to maintain an adequate fluid intake to facilitate the uric acid excretion.
- Tell patient to avoid exposure to persons with infections.
- Advise patient that hair should grow back after therapy has ended.
- Tell patient to report a sore throat, fever, or any unusual bruising or bleeding.

uracil mustard
Pregnancy risk category: D

How supplied
Capsules: 1 mg

Indications, route, and dosage
Indications and dosage may vary. Check current literature for recommended protocol.
Chronic lymphocytic and myelocytic leukemia; Hodgkin's disease; non-Hodgkin's lymphomas of the histiocytic and lymphocytic types; reticulum cell sarcoma; lymphomas; mycosis fungoides; polycythemia vera; ovarian, cervical, and lung cancers
Adults: 1 to 2 mg P.O. daily for 3 months or until desired response or toxicity occurs; maintenance dosage is 1 mg daily for 3 out of 4 weeks until optimum response or relapse occurs. Alternatively, 3 to 5 mg P.O. for 7 days, not to exceed a total dose of 0.5 mg/kg, followed by 1 mg daily until response occurs, then 1 mg daily 3 out of 4 weeks; or 0.15 mg/kg P.O. once weekly for 4 weeks.
Children: 0.3 mg/kg P.O. weekly for 4 weeks.

Thrombocytosis
Adults: 1 to 2 mg P.O. daily for 14 days.

Pharmacodynamics

Uracil mustard exerts its cytotoxic activity by cross-linking strands of DNA, interfering with DNA and RNA replication and disrupting normal nucleic acid function, resulting in cell death.

Pharmacokinetics

Absorption: In animal studies, uracil mustard is absorbed quickly but incompletely after oral administration.
Distribution: Unknown.
Metabolism: Unknown.
Excretion: In studies using dogs, elimination of uracil mustard from the plasma is rapid, with no drug detected 2 hours after administration. Less than 1% of a dose is excreted unchanged in urine.

Contraindications and precautions

Uracil mustard is contraindicated in patients with a history of hypersensitivity to tartrazine, a dye contained in the capsules. The incidence of hypersensitivity is low, but it seems to occur frequently in patients allergic to aspirin.

Uracil mustard should be used cautiously in patients whose bone marrow shows infiltration with malignant cells, because hematopoietic toxicity may be increased.

Interactions

None reported.

Effects on diagnostic tests

Uracil mustard therapy may increase blood and urine uric acid levels.

Adverse reactions

CNS: irritability, nervousness, mental cloudiness, depression.
DERM: pruritus, dermatitis, hyperpigmentation.
GI: nausea, vomiting, diarrhea, epigastric distress, abdominal pain, anorexia.

Canada only   †Off-label use   Italicized adverse reactions are life-threatening.

HEMA: *bone-marrow depression* (dose-limiting), *thrombocytopenia, leukopenia,* anemia.
Metabolic: hyperuricemia.
Other: alopecia.

Overdose and treatment

Clinical manifestations of overdose include myelosuppression, nausea, and vomiting.

Treatment is usually supportive and includes antiemetics and transfusion of blood components.

Special considerations

Besides those relevant to all alkylating agents, consider the following recommendations.
- Give at bedtime to reduce nausea.
- Drug is usually not administered until 2 or 3 weeks after the maximum effect of previous drugs is reached or until radiation effects are evident.
- Watch for signs of ecchymoses, easy bruising, and petechiae.
- To prevent hyperuricemia and resulting uric acid nephropathy, allopurinol can be given; keep patient hydrated. Monitor uric acid levels.
- Monitor platelet count regularly. Perform a CBC one to two times weekly for 4 weeks, then 4 weeks after stopping drug.
- Avoid all I.M. injections when platelet count is below 100,000/mm^3.
- Anticoagulants and aspirin products should be used cautiously. Watch closely for signs of bleeding. Also instruct patient to avoid nonprescription products containing aspirin.
- Dose modification may be required in severe thrombocytopenia, aplastic anemia or leukopenia, or in acute leukemia.

Information for the patient
- Emphasize the importance of continuing the medication despite nausea and vomiting.

- Tell patient to call immediately if vomiting occurs shortly after taking a dose, if he develops a sore throat or fever, or if he notices unusual bruising or bleeding.
- Encourage adequate fluid intake to increase urine output and facilitate excretion of uric acid. Patient should void frequently.
- Tell patient that hair growth should resume after treatment has ended.
- Advise patient to avoid exposure to persons with infections.

Antibiotic antineoplastics

bleomycin sulfate	mitoxantrone hydrochloride
dactinomycin	pentostatin
daunorubicin hydrochloride	plicamycin
doxorubicin hydrochloride	procarbazine hydrochloride
idarubicin hydrochloride	streptozocin
mitomycin	

Although these agents are classified as antibiotics, the toxicity associated with them rules out their use as antimicrobial agents. These agents interfere with proliferation of malignant cells through several mechanisms. Their action may be cell-cycle nonspecific, cell-cycle specific, or both. Some antibiotic antineoplastics even demonstrate activity that resembles alkylating agents or antimetabolites; for example, streptozocin is considered an alkylating agent because of its therapeutic activity.

Pharmacology

By binding to or complexing with DNA, antineoplastic antibiotics inhibit DNA and RNA synthesis. They do so by one of the following mechanisms: They inhibit DNA-dependent RNA synthesis, directly inhibit RNA synthesis, alter DNA and thus inhibit RNA synthesis, or react with DNA to cause strand breakage.

Clinical indications and actions

Antibiotic antineoplastics are useful alone or in combination with other types of antineoplastic agents for treating various tumors. For the specific uses, see the individual drug entries discussed in this chapter.

Overview of adverse reactions

The most frequent adverse reactions to the antibiotic antineoplastic agents include nausea, vomiting, diarrhea, fever, chills, sore throat, anxiety, confusion, flank or joint pain, swelling of feet or lower legs, hair loss, redness or pain at injection site, bone marrow depression, and leukopenia.

Special considerations

- Vital signs and patency of catheter or I.V. line should be monitored throughout administration.
- Carefully follow all established procedures for the safe and proper handling, administration, and disposal of chemotherapeutic drugs.
- Treat extravasation promptly.
- Attempt to ease anxiety in patient and family before treatment.
- Monitor BUN, hematocrit level, platelet count, ALT (formerly SGPT), AST (formerly SGOT), LDH, serum bilirubin, serum creatinine, uric acid, and total and differential WBC counts.
- Avoid immunizations if possible. Warn patient to avoid close contact with persons who have taken the oral poliovirus vaccine.

Information for the patient

- Tell patient to avoid exposure to persons with bacterial or viral infections because chemotherapy can make the patient more susceptible to infection. Urge him to report infection immediately.
- Advise patient to use proper hygiene and caution when using toothbrush, dental floss, and toothpicks. Chemo-

therapy can increase incidence of microbial infection, delayed healing, and bleeding gums.
- Tell patient that dental work should be completed before therapy begins, if possible, or delayed until blood counts are normal.
- Warn patient that he may bruise easily because of drug's effects on blood counts.
- Tell patient to immediately report redness, pain, or swelling at injection site. Local tissue injury and scarring may result if I.V. infiltrates.

bleomycin sulfate
Blenoxane

Pregnancy risk category: D

How supplied

Injection: 15-unit ampules (1 unit = 1 mg)

Indications, route, and dosage

Indications and dosage may vary. Check literature for current protocol.
Hodgkin's disease, squamous cell carcinoma, non-Hodgkin's lymphoma, or testicular cancer
Adults: 10 to 20 units/m² (0.25 to 0.5 units/kg) I.V., I.M., or S.C., once or twice weekly. After 50% response, maintenance dose of 1 unit daily or 5 units weekly.
†**Malignant pleural effusion**
Adults: 50 to 60 units by intracavitary administration.

Pharmacodynamics

The exact mechanism of bleomycin's cytotoxicity is unknown. Its action may be through scission of single- and double-stranded DNA and inhibition of DNA, RNA, and protein synthesis. Bleomycin also appears to inhibit cell progression out of the G_2 phase.

Pharmacokinetics

Absorption: Bleomycin is poorly absorbed across the GI tract following oral administration. I.M. administration results in lower serum levels than those occurring after equivalent I.V. doses.

Distribution: Bleomycin distributes widely into total body water, mainly in the skin, lungs, kidneys, peritoneum, and lymphatic tissue.

Metabolism: The metabolic fate of bleomycin is undetermined; however, extensive tissue inactivation occurs in the liver and kidney and much less in the skin and lungs.

Excretion: Bleomycin and its metabolites are excreted primarily in urine. The terminal plasma elimination phase half-life is reported at 2 hours.

Contraindications and precautions

Bleomycin is contraindicated in patients with a history of hypersensitivity or idiosyncratic reaction to the drug.

Use with caution in patients with renal impairment because drug accumulation may occur. Also use cautiously in patients with pulmonary impairment; monitor the patient carefully for signs of pulmonary toxicity because pulmonary fibrosis may occur. Patient should have chest X-rays every 1 to 2 weeks during therapy and evaluation of pulmonary diffusion capacity for carbon dioxide every month.

Interactions

Concomitant use with phenytoin or digoxin may decrease serum levels of those agents.

Effects on diagnostic tests

Bleomycin therapy may increase blood and urine concentrations of uric acid.

Adverse reactions

CNS: hyperesthesia of scalp and fingers, headache.
DERM: erythema, vesiculation, and hardening and discoloration of palmar and plantar skin in about 8% of patients; desquamation of hands, feet, and pressure areas; hyperpigmentation; acne.

GI: stomatitis, prolonged anorexia in approximately 13% of patients, nausea, vomiting, diarrhea.

Respiratory: fine crackles, fever, dyspnea, nonproductive cough; *dose-limiting pulmonary fibrosis* in about 10% of patients. (*Note:* Drug should be discontinued if patient develops signs of pulmonary fibrosis or mucocutaneous toxicity.)

Other: reversible alopecia, swelling of interphalangeal joints, leukocytosis, *allergic reaction* (fever up to 106° F [41.1° C] with chills up to 5 hours after injection; *anaphylaxis* in approximately 1% to 6% of patients).

Overdose and treatment

Clinical manifestations of overdose include pulmonary fibrosis, fever, chills, vesiculation, and hyperpigmentation.

Treatment is usually supportive and includes antipyretics for fever.

Special considerations

- To prepare solution for I.M. administration, reconstitute the drug with 1 to 5 ml of 0.9% sodium chloride solution, sterile water for injection, or dextrose 5% in water.
- For I.V. administration, dilute with a minimum of 5 ml of diluent and administer over 10 minutes as I.V. push injection.
- Prepare infusions of bleomycin in glass bottles because absorption of drug to plastic occurs with time. Plastic syringes do not interfere with bleomycin activity.
- Wear gloves and wash hands when preparing and administering bleomycin.
- Bleomycin can be administered by intracavitary, intra-arterial, or intratumor injection. It can also be instilled into the bladder for bladder tumors.
- Cumulative lifetime dosage should not exceed 400 units.
- Response to therapy may take 2 to 3 weeks.
- Administer a 1-unit test dose before therapy to assess hypersensitivity to bleomycin. If no reaction occurs, then follow the dosing schedule. The test dose can be incorporated as part of the total dose for the regimen.
- Have epinephrine, diphenhydramine, I.V. corticosteroids, and oxygen available in case of anaphylactic reaction.

---

*Canada only   †Off-label use   Italicized adverse reactions are life-threatening.

- Premedication with aspirin, steroids, and diphenhydramine may reduce drug fever and risk of anaphylaxis.
- Dosage should be reduced in patients with renal or pulmonary impairment.
- Drug concentrates in keratin of squamous epithelium. To prevent linear streaking, don't use adhesive dressings on skin.
- Allergic reactions may be delayed, especially in patients with lymphoma.
- Pulmonary function tests should be performed to establish a baseline and then monitored periodically. They also may be useful in predicting pulmonary fibrosis.
- Monitor chest X-rays, and auscultate the lungs.
- Bleomycin is stable for 24 hours at room temperature and 48 hours under refrigeration. Refrigerate unopened vials containing dry powder.

Information for the patient
Explain that hair should grow back after treatment is discontinued.

Geriatric use
Use with caution in patients over age 70. They are at increased risk for pulmonary toxicity.

dactinomycin (actinomycin D)
Cosmegen
Pregnancy risk category: C

How supplied
Injectable: 500-mcg vial

Indications, route, and dosage
Indications and dosage may vary. Check current literature for recommended protocol.
Melanomas, sarcomas, trophoblastic tumors in women, testicular cancer
Adults: 10 to 15 mcg/kg I.V. for a maximum of 5 days q 4 to 6 weeks, or 500 mcg/m^2 I.V. once a week (maximum of 2 mg/week) for 3 weeks. Alternatively, for isolation-perfusion,

use 50 mcg/kg for lower extremity or pelvis; for upper extremity, 35 mcg/kg.

Wilms' tumor, rhabdomyosarcoma, Ewing's sarcoma
Children: 10 to 15 mcg/kg/day or 450 mcg/m^2/day I.V. (maximum dose: 500 mcg/day for 5 days or 2.4 mg/m^2 in divided doses over 7 days). If all signs of toxicity have disappeared, may be repeated in 4 to 6 weeks.

Note: Use body surface area calculation in obese or edematous patients. (See "Calculating body surface area" in the Appendices for more information.)

Pharmacodynamics

Dactinomycin exerts its cytotoxic activity by intercalating between DNA base pairs and uncoiling the DNA helix. The result is inhibition of DNA synthesis and DNA-dependent RNA synthesis.

Pharmacokinetics

Absorption: Due to its vesicant properties, dactinomycin must be administered I.V.
Distribution: Dactinomycin is widely distributed into body tissues, with the highest levels found in the bone marrow and nucleated cells. The drug does not cross the blood-brain barrier to any significant extent.
Metabolism: Dactinomycin is only minimally metabolized in the liver.
Excretion: Dactinomycin and its metabolites are excreted in the urine and bile. The plasma elimination half-life of the drug is 36 hours.

Contraindications and precautions

Dactinomycin is contraindicated in patients who are infected with chicken pox or herpes zoster because of risk of serious generalized disease and death. Drug should be used during pregnancy only when potential benefits to the mother outweigh risks to the fetus.

Use with extreme caution in patients with renal, hepatic, or bone marrow impairment and viral infections. Use cautiously in metastatic testicular tumors, in combination with chlorambucil and methotrexate therapy. Extreme bone marrow and GI toxicity can occur with this combined therapy.

Also use cautiously in patients who have received cytotoxic drugs or radiation therapy within 6 weeks or in patients with a history of gout, infection, or hematologic compromise, because of increased potential for adverse effects.

Interactions

None reported.

Effects on diagnostic tests

Dactinomycin therapy may increase blood and urine concentrations of uric acid.

Adverse reactions

Bone marrow depression and GI reactions are the dose-limiting toxicity factors.

DERM: erythema; desquamation; hyperpigmentation of skin, especially in previously irradiated areas; acnelike eruptions (reversible).

GI: anorexia, nausea, vomiting, abdominal pain, diarrhea, stomatitis, esophagitis, pharyngitis. (*Note:* Drug should be discontinued if diarrhea and stomatitis develop. Therapy may resume when these conditions subside.)

HEMA: anemia, *leukopenia, thrombocytopenia, pancytopenia, agranulocytosis.*

Local: phlebitis, severe damage to soft tissue.

Other: reversible alopecia, hepatotoxicity.

Overdose and treatment

Clinical manifestations of overdose include myelosuppression, nausea, vomiting, glossitis, and oral ulceration.

Treatment is generally supportive and includes antiemetics and transfusion of blood components.

Special considerations

• To reconstitute for I.V. administration, add 1.1 ml of sterile water for injection to drug to give a concentration of 0.5 mg/ml. Do not use a preserved diluent because precipitation may occur.
• Use gloves when preparing and administering this drug.

- May dilute further with dextrose 5% in water or 0.9% sodium chloride solution for administration by I.V. infusion.
- Discard any unused solution because it doesn't contain any preservatives.
- May administer by I.V. push injection into the tubing of a free-flowing I.V. infusion. Do not administer through an in-line I.V. filter.
- Treatment of extravasation includes topical administration of dimethyl sulfoxide and cold compresses.
- To reduce nausea, give antiemetic before administering. Nausea usually occurs within 30 minutes of a dose.
- Monitor CBC daily and platelet counts every third day. Observe for signs of bleeding.
- Monitor renal and hepatic functions.
- Patients who have received other cytotoxic drugs or radiation within 6 weeks of dactinomycin may exhibit erythema, followed by hyperpigmentation or edema, or both; desquamation; vesiculation; and, rarely, necrosis.

Information for the patient
- Advise patient to avoid exposure to persons with infections.
- Warn patient that alopecia may occur but is usually reversible.
- Tell patient to promptly report sore throat, fever, or any signs of bleeding.

daunorubicin hydrochloride
Cerubidine
Pregnancy risk category: D

How supplied
Injection: 20-mg vials

Indications, route, and dosage
Indications and dosage may vary. Check current literature for recommended protocol.

Remission induction in acute nonlymphocytic leukemia (myelogenous, monocytic, erythroid)

Adults: As a single agent—30 to 60 mg/m² I.V. daily on days 1, 2, and 3 q 3 to 4 weeks; or 800 mcg to 1 mg/kg for 3 to 6 days, repeated q 3 to 4 weeks. Maximum dosage is 550 mg/m² (450 mg/m² for patients who have received chest irradiation). In combination—25 to 45 mg/m² I.V. daily on days 1, 2, and 3 of the first course and on days 1 and 2 of subsequent courses with cytosine arabinoside infusions.

Adults age 60 and over: Initially, 30 mg/m² I.V. daily for 3 days. Repeat courses q 3 to 4 weeks with 30 mg/m² daily for 2 days.

Children: 25 mg/m² weekly, usually combined with vincristine and prednisone.

Note: Dose should be reduced if hepatic function is impaired.

Pharmacodynamics

Daunorubicin exerts its cytotoxic activity by intercalating between DNA base pairs, uncoiling the DNA helix, and inhibiting DNA synthesis and DNA-dependent RNA synthesis. The drug may also inhibit polymerase activity.

Pharmacokinetics

Absorption: Because of its vesicant nature, daunorubicin must be given I.V.

Distribution: Daunorubicin is widely distributed into body tissues, with the highest concentrations found in the spleen, kidneys, liver, lungs, and heart. The drug does not cross the blood-brain barrier.

Metabolism: The drug is extensively metabolized in the liver by microsomal enzymes. One of the metabolites has cytotoxic activity.

Excretion: Daunorubicin and its metabolites are primarily excreted in bile, with a small portion excreted in urine. Plasma elimination has been described as biphasic, with an initial phase half-life of about 45 minutes and a terminal phase half-life of about 18¹/₂ hours.

Contraindications and precautions

Daunorubicin is contraindicated in patients with life-threatening myelosuppression, preexisting cardiac disease, severe

---

infections, or hepatic or renal dysfunction because drug may worsen these conditions. The drug should not be given to pregnant patients because of significant risk to the fetus. Use cautiously in patients with moderate hepatic, renal, cardiac, or bone marrow dysfunction.

Interactions

When used concomitantly, other hepatotoxic drugs may increase the risk of hepatotoxicity with daunorubicin.

Do not mix daunorubicin with either heparin sodium or dexamethasone phosphate. Admixture of these agents results in the formation of a precipitate.

Effects on diagnostic tests

Daunorubicin therapy may increase blood and urine concentrations of uric acid.

Daunorubicin therapy may also cause an increase in serum alkaline phosphatase, AST (formerly SGOT), and bilirubin levels, indicating drug-induced hepatotoxicity.

Adverse reactions

CV: *irreversible cardiomyopathy* (dose-related), ECG changes, arrhythmias, *pericarditis, myocarditis*. (*Note:* Drug should be discontinued if patient develops signs of CHF or cardiomyopathy.)
DERM: rash.
GI: nausea, vomiting, stomatitis, esophagitis, anorexia, diarrhea.
GU: nephrotoxicity, transient red urine.
HEMA: *bone marrow depression* (dose-limiting), anemia, *pancytopenia* (nadir between 10 and 14 days), *leukopenia, thrombocytopenia*.
Hepatic: hepatotoxicity.
Metabolic: hyperuricemia.
Local: severe cellulitis or tissue sloughing if drug extravasates.
Other: generalized alopecia, fever, chills.

Overdose and treatment

Clinical manifestations of overdose include myelosuppression, nausea, vomiting, and stomatitis.

Treatment is usually supportive and includes transfusion of blood components and administration of antiemetics.

Special considerations

- To reconstitute the drug for I.V. administration, add 4 ml of sterile water for injection to a 20-mg vial to give a concentration of 5 mg/ml.
- Drug may be diluted further into 100 ml of dextrose 5% in water or 0.9% sodium chloride solution and infused over 30 to 45 minutes.
- For I.V. push administration, withdraw reconstituted drug into a syringe containing 10 to 15 ml of 0.9% sodium chloride solution, and inject over 2 to 3 minutes into the tubing of a free-flowing I.V. infusion. Reconstituted solution is stable for 24 hours at room temperature.
- Reddish color of drug is similar to that of doxorubicin. Do not confuse the two drugs.
- Erythematous streaking along the vein or flushing in the face indicates too-rapid administration.
- Extravasation may be treated with ice packs to the site.
- Antiemetics may be used to prevent or treat nausea and vomiting.
- Darkness or redness of the skin may occur in prior radiation fields.
- To prevent cardiomyopathy, cumulative dose should be limited to 550 mg/m^2 (450 mg/m^2 when patient has been receiving any other cardiotoxic agent, such as cyclophosphamide, or radiation therapy that encompasses the heart).
- Dosage should be reduced in patients with hepatic or renal impairment; in patients with serum bilirubin of 1.2 to 3 mg/dl, reduce dose by 25%; with serum bilirubin or creatinine levels over 3 mg/dl, reduce dose by 50%.
- Monitor ECG before treatment and monthly during treatment.
- Monitor CBC and hepatic function.
- Note if resting pulse rate is high (a sign of cardiac adverse reactions).
- Do not use a scalp tourniquet or apply ice to prevent alopecia because this may compromise the drug's effectiveness.

- Nausea and vomiting may be very severe and last 24 to 48 hours.

Information for the patient
- Warn patient that urine may be red for 1 to 2 days and that this is a drug effect, not evidence of bleeding.
- Advise patient that alopecia may occur, but is usually reversible.
- Tell patient to avoid exposure to persons with infections.
- Encourage adequate fluid intake to increase urine output and facilitate uric acid excretion.
- Warn patient that nausea and vomiting may be severe and may last for 24 to 48 hours.
- Tell patient to report a sore throat, fever, or any signs of bleeding.

Geriatric use
- Elderly patients have an increased incidence of drug-induced cardiotoxicity.
- Be sure to monitor for hematologic toxicity because some elderly patients have poor bone marrow reserve.

doxorubicin hydrochloride
Adriamycin PFS, Adriamycin RDF
Pregnancy risk category: D

How supplied

Injection: 10-mg, 20-mg, 50-mg, 100-mg, 150-mg vials
Injection (preservative-free): 2 mg/ml

Indications, route, and dosage

Indications and dosage may vary. Check current literature for recommended protocol.

Cancer of bladder, kidney, breast, cervix, head, neck, liver, lungs, ovary, prostate gland, stomach, testicles, brain, or blood and lymph system; sarcomas

Adults: 60 to 75 mg/m² I.V. as a single dose q 3 weeks; or 25 to 30 mg/m² I.V. as a single daily dose on days 1 to 3 of 4-week cycle. Alternatively, 20 mg/m² I.V. once weekly. Maximum cumulative dosage is 550 mg/m^2 (450 mg/m^2 in patients who have received chest irradiation).

Children: 30 mg/m^2 I.V. as single daily dose on days 1 to 3 of 4-week cycle.

Pharmacodynamics

Doxorubicin exerts its cytotoxic activity by intercalating between DNA base pairs and uncoiling the DNA helix. The result is inhibition of DNA synthesis and DNA-dependent RNA synthesis. Doxorubicin also inhibits protein synthesis.

Pharmacokinetics

Absorption: Because of its vesicant effects, doxorubicin must be administered I.V.

Distribution: Doxorubicin distributes widely into body tissues, with the highest concentrations found in the liver, heart, and kidneys. The drug does not cross the blood-brain barrier.

Metabolism: Doxorubicin is extensively metabolized by hepatic microsomal enzymes to several metabolites, one of which possesses cytotoxic activity.

Excretion: Doxorubicin and its metabolites are excreted primarily in bile. A minute amount is eliminated in urine. The plasma elimination of doxorubicin is described as biphasic, with a half-life of about $1/2$ hour in the initial phase and $16^1/_2$ hours in the terminal phase.

Contraindications and precautions

Doxorubicin is contraindicated in patients with hepatic dysfunction, depressed bone marrow function, or impaired cardiac function and in patients who have previously received lifetime cumulative doses of doxorubicin or daunorubicin because of increased potential for cardiac or hematopoietic toxicity.

Interactions

Concomitant use with streptozocin may increase the plasma half-life of doxorubicin by an unknown mechanism, increasing the drug's activity. Concomitant use of daunorubicin or cyclophosphamide may potentiate the cardiotoxicity of doxorubicin through additive effects on the heart.

Doxorubicin should not be mixed with heparin sodium, fluorouracil, aminophylline, cephalosporins, dexamethasone phosphate, or hydrocortisone sodium phosphate because a precipitate will form. Serum digoxin levels may be decreased if used concomitantly with doxorubicin.

Effects on diagnostic tests

Doxorubicin therapy may increase blood and urine concentrations of uric acid.

Adverse reactions

CV: *cardiotoxicity,* seen in such ECG changes as sinus tachycardia, T-wave flattening, ST-segment depression, and voltage reduction; *arrhythmias; irreversible cardiomyopathy,* sometimes with pulmonary edema.
DERM: hyperpigmentation, especially in previously irradiated areas.
GI: nausea, vomiting, diarrhea, stomatitis, esophagitis.
GU: transient red urine.
HEMA: *leukopenia,* especially agranulocytosis, during days 10 to 15, with recovery by day 21; *thrombocytopenia; bone marrow depression* (dose-limiting). *Note:* Drug should be discontinued if hematopoietic toxicity becomes severe.
Local: severe cellulitis.
Other: hyperpigmentation of nails and dermal creases, complete alopecia.

Overdose and treatment

Clinical manifestations of overdose include myelosuppression, nausea, vomiting, mucositis, and irreversible myocardial toxicity.

Treatment is usually supportive and includes transfusion of blood components; administration of antiemetics, antibiotics for infections that may develop, and digitalis preparations; and symptomatic treatment of mucositis.

Special considerations

• To reconstitute, add 5 ml of 0.9% sodium chloride solution to the 10-mg vial, 10 ml to the 20-mg vial, and 25 ml to the 50-mg vial, to yield a concentration of 2 mg/ml.

- Doxorubicin may be further diluted with 0.9% sodium chloride solution or dextrose 5% in water and administered by I.V. infusion.
- Doxorubicin may be administered by I.V. push injection over 5 to 10 minutes into the tubing of a free-flowing I.V. infusion.
- The alternative dosage schedule (once-weekly dosing) has been found to cause a lower incidence of cardiomyopathy.
- When cumulative dose exceeds 550 mg/m^2 body surface area, about 30% of patients develop cardiac adverse reactions, which begin 2 weeks to 6 months after stopping the drug.
- Children under age 2 have a higher incidence of drug-induced cardiotoxicity.
- Streaking along a vein or facial flushing indicates that the drug is being administered too rapidly.
- Applying a scalp tourniquet or ice may decrease alopecia. However, never use these items when treating leukemias or other neoplasms in which tumor stem cells may be present in the scalp.
- Doxorubicin should be discontinued or rate of infusion slowed if tachycardia develops.
- Treat extravasation with ice packs.
- Monitor CBC and hepatic function.
- Decrease dosage as follows if serum bilirubin level increases: 50% of dose when bilirubin level is 1.2 to 3 mg/100 ml; 25% of dose when bilirubin level exceeds 3 mg/100 ml.
- Esophagitis is very common in patients who have also received radiation therapy.

Information for the patient
- Encourage adequate fluid intake to increase urine output and facilitate uric acid excretion.
- Advise patient to avoid exposure to persons with infections.
- Warn patient that alopecia will occur. Explain that hair growth should resume 2 to 5 months after drug is stopped.
- Advise patient that urine will become reddish for 1 to 2 days after the dose and does not indicate bleeding. The urine may also stain clothes.

- Tell patient not to receive any immunizations during therapy and for several weeks afterward. Other members of the patient's household should also not receive immunizations during the same period.
- Tell patient to report unusual bruising or bleeding promptly.

Geriatric use

Patients over age 70 have an increased incidence of drug-induced cardiotoxicity. Caution should be taken in elderly patients with low bone marrow reserve to prevent serious hematologic toxicity.

idarubicin hydrochloride
Idamycin

Pregnancy risk category: D

How supplied

Injection: 5 mg, 10 mg (lyophilized powder) in single-dose vials with 50 or 100 mg lactose

Indications, route, and dosage

Indications and dosage may vary. Check current literature for recommended protocol.

Acute myelocytic leukemia in adults, including French-American-British classifications M1 through M7, in combination with other approved antileukemic agents

Adults: 12 mg/m² daily by slow I.V. injection (over 10 to 15 minutes) for 3 days in combination with 100 mg/m² of cytarabine given daily by continuous infusion for 7 days or as a 25-mg/m² bolus followed by 200 mg/m² by continuous I.V. infusion daily for 5 days.

A second course may be administered if needed. If patient experiences severe mucositis, delay administration until recovery is complete and reduce dosage by 25%. Also reduce dosage in patients with hepatic or renal impairment. Idarubicin should not be given if bilirubin level is above 5 mg/dl.

Pharmacodynamics

Idarubicin inhibits nucleic acid synthesis by intercalation and interacts with the enzyme topoisomerase II. It is highly lipophilic, which results in an increased rate of cellular uptake.

Pharmacokinetics

Absorption: Peak cellular concentrations are achieved within minutes of I.V. injection.

Distribution: Idarubicin is highly lipophilic and excessively tissue-bound (about 97%), with highest concentrations in nucleated blood and bone marrow cells. Its metabolite, idarubicinol, is detected in CSF; the clinical significance of this is under evaluation.

Metabolism: Extensive extrahepatic metabolism is indicated. Metabolite has cytotoxic activity.

Excretion: Predominantly by biliary excretion as its metabolite and, to a lesser extent, by renal elimination. The mean terminal half-life is 22 hours (range, 4 to 46 hours) when used as a single agent and 20 hours (range, 7 to 38 hours) when combined with cytarabine. Plasma levels of metabolite are sustained for longer than 8 days.

Contraindications and precautions

Idarubicin is contraindicated in patients with severe myelosuppression, preexisting cardiac disease, severe hemorrhagic conditions, or overwhelming infection.

Use with extreme caution in hepatic or renal function impairment. Reduce dosage.

Interactions

Idarubicin should not be mixed with other drugs unless specific compatibility data are available. Heparin causes precipitation. Degradation occurs with prolonged contact with alkaline solutions.

Effects on diagnostic tests

No direct laboratory test interference has been reported. However, drug-induced hepatic, renal, and bone marrow toxicity may occur.

Adverse reactions

CNS: headache, changed mental status, seizures.

CV: *CHF,* atrial fibrillation, chest pain, *MI,* asymptomatic decline in left ventricular ejection fraction, myocardial insufficiency, *arrhythmias,* hemorrhage, myocardial toxicity.

DERM: alopecia, rash, urticaria, bullous erythrodermatous rash of palms and soles, hives at injection site.

GI: nausea, vomiting, cramps, diarrhea, mucositis, severe enterocolitis with perforation (rare).

HEMA: *severe bone marrow depression.*

Respiratory: pulmonary allergy.

Other: infection, fever, changes in hepatic and renal functions, aplasia, local tissue necrosis (if extravasation occurs).

Overdose and treatment

Severe and prolonged myelosuppression and possibly increased severity of GI toxicity is anticipated. Supportive treatment, including platelet transfusions, antibiotics, and treatment of mucositis, is required. Acute cardiac toxicity with severe arrhythmias and delayed cardiac failure may also occur. Peritoneal dialysis or hemodialysis is not effective.

Special considerations

- Frequently monitor hepatic and renal function and CBC.
- Hyperuricemia may result from rapid lysis of leukemic cells; take appropriate preventive measures (including adequate hydration) before starting treatment.
- Control systemic infections before therapy.
- Administer over 10 to 15 minutes into a free-flowing I.V. infusion of 0.9% sodium chloride solution or dextrose 5% in water, which is running into a large vein.
- If extravasation or signs of extravasation occur, discontinue infusion immediately and restart in another vein. Treat with intermittent ice packs—$^1/_2$ hour immediately, then $^1/_2$ hour q.i.d. for 4 days—and evaluate affected extremity.
- Prevent or treat nausea and vomiting with antiemetics.
- Reconstitute, using 5 or 10 ml of 0.9% sodium chloride solution, for the 5- or 10-mg vial respectively, to give a final

concentration of 1 mg/ml. Do not use bacteriostatic sodium chloride solution.
• Follow usual chemotherapy mixing precautions. Vial is under negative pressure.
• Reconstituted solutions are stable for 3 days (72 hours) at room temperature (59° to 86° F [15° to 30° C]); for 7 days, if refrigerated. Discard unused solutions appropriately.

Information for the patient
• Instruct patient how to recognize signs and symptoms of extravasation and to notify doctor or nurse promptly if these occur.
• Tell patient to report signs and symptoms of infection, including persistent fever or sore throat.
• Tell patient to minimize dangerous behavior that can cause bleeding and to report any bleeding or abnormal bruising.

mitomycin (mitomycin C; MTC)
Mutamycin
Pregnancy risk category: C

How supplied

Injection: 5-mg, 20-mg, 40-mg vials

Indications, route, and dosage

Indications and dosage may vary. Check current literature for recommended protocol.
Stomach, pancreatic, breast, colon, head, neck, lung, and hepatic cancers
Adults: 2 mg/m² I.V. daily for 5 days. Stop drug for 2 days, then repeat dose for 5 more days; or 10 to 20 mg/m² as a single dose. Repeat cycle q 6 to 8 weeks. Stop drug if WBC count is below 3,000/mm³ or platelet count is below 75,000/mm³.

Pharmacodynamics

Mitomycin exerts its cytotoxic activity by a mechanism similar to that of the alkylating agents. The drug is converted to an active compound that forms cross-links between strands of DNA, thereby inhibiting DNA synthesis. Mitomycin also inhibits RNA and protein synthesis to a lesser extent.

Pharmacokinetics

Absorption: Because of its vesicant nature, mitomycin must be administered I.V.

Distribution: Mitomycin distributes widely into body tissues; animal studies show that the highest concentrations are found in the muscle, eyes, lungs, intestines, and stomach. The drug does not cross the blood-brain barrier.

Metabolism: Mitomycin is metabolized by hepatic microsomal enzymes and is also deactivated in the kidneys, spleen, brain, and heart.

Excretion: Mitomycin and its metabolites are excreted in urine. A small portion is eliminated in bile and feces.

Contraindications and precautions

Mitomycin is contraindicated in patients with a history of hypersensitivity to the drug; in patients with a WBC count below 3,000/mm^3, platelet count below 75,000/mm^3, or serum creatinine level above 1.7 mg/100 ml; and in those with coagulation disorders, prolonged prothrombin time, or serious infections, because of the potential for adverse effects.

Interactions

Concomitant use with dextran and urokinase enhances the cytotoxic activity of mitomycin. Through a series of enzymatic processes, these agents increase autolysis of cells, adding to the cell death caused by mitomycin.

Effects on diagnostic tests

Mitomycin therapy, through drug-induced renal toxicity, may increase serum creatinine and BUN concentrations.

Adverse reactions

CNS: paresthesias.
GI: nausea, vomiting, anorexia, stomatitis.

HEMA: *bone marrow depression* (dose-limiting), *thrombocytopenia, leukopenia* (may be delayed up to 8 weeks and may be cumulative with successive doses). *Note:* Drug should be discontinued if WBC count is below 3,000/mm³ or platelet count is below 75,000/mm³.

Local: desquamation, induration, pruritus, pain at site of injection; with extravasation: cellulitis, ulceration, sloughing.

Other: reversible alopecia; purple coloration of nail beds; fever; syndrome characterized by microangiopathic hemolytic anemia, *thrombocytopenia*, renal toxicity, and hypertension.

Overdose and treatment

Clinical manifestations of overdose include myelosuppression, nausea, vomiting, and alopecia.

Treatment is usually supportive and includes transfusion of blood components, administration of antiemetics, and administration of antibiotics for any infections that develop.

Special considerations

• To reconstitute, add 10 ml of sterile water for injection to the 5-mg vial, and 40 ml to the 20-mg vial, to give a concentration of 0.5 mg/ml.

• Mitomycin may be administered by I.V. push injection slowly over 5 to 10 minutes into the tubing of a free-flowing I.V. infusion.

• Mitomycin can be further diluted to 100 to 150 ml with 0.9% sodium chloride solution or dextrose 5% in water for I.V. infusion (over 30 to 60 minutes or longer).

• Reconstituted solution remains stable for 1 week at room temperature and for 2 weeks if refrigerated.

• Mitomycin has been administered intra-arterially to treat certain tumors; for example, into the hepatic artery for colon cancer. It has also been given as a continuous daily infusion.

• An off-label use of this drug is to treat small bladder papillomas. It is instilled directly into the bladder in a concentration of 1 mg/ml in 20 ml of sterile water.

• Ulcers caused by extravasation develop late and dorsal to the extravasation site. Apply cold compresses for at least 12 hours.

• Continue CBC and blood studies at least 7 weeks after therapy is stopped. Monitor for signs of bleeding.

Information for the patient
• Tell patient to avoid exposure to persons with infections.
• Warn patient not to receive immunizations during therapy and for several weeks afterward. Members of the patient's household should not receive immunizations during the same period.
• Reassure patient that hair should grow back after treatment has been discontinued.
• Tell patient to call promptly if he develops a sore throat or fever or notices any unusual bruising or bleeding.

mitoxantrone hydrochloride
Novantrone

Pregnancy risk category: D

How supplied

Injection: 2 mg mitoxantrone base/ml in 10-ml, 12.5-ml, 15-ml vials

Indications, route, and dosage

Indications and dosage may vary. Check current literature for recommended protocol.
Initial treatment in combination with other approved drugs for acute nonlymphocytic leukemia
Adults: For induction (in combination chemotherapy), 12 mg/m^2 daily by I.V. infusion on days 1 to 3, and 100 mg/m^2 of cytarabine by continuous I.V. infusion (over 24 hours) on days 1 to 7 for 7 days.

Most complete remissions follow initial course of induction therapy. A second course may be given if antileukemic response is incomplete: give mitoxantrone for 2 days and cytarabine for 5 days using the same daily dosage levels. Second course of therapy should be withheld until toxicity clears if severe or life-threatening nonhematologic toxicity occurs.

Pharmacodynamics

Mitoxantrone's mechanism of action is not completely established. It is a DNA-reactive agent that has cytocidal effects on proliferating and nonproliferating cells, suggestive of lack of cell-cycle specificity.

Pharmacokinetics

Absorption: Not applicable. Administered only by I.V. infusion.
Distribution: Mitoxantrone is about 78% plasma protein-bound.
Metabolism: Metabolized by the liver.
Excretion: Excretion is through the renal and hepatobiliary systems. Approximately 6% to 11% of dose is excreted in urine within 5 days: about 65% as unchanged drug, 35% as two inactive metabolites. Within 5 days, about 25% of dose is excreted in feces.

Contraindications and precautions

Mitoxantrone is contraindicated in patients with known hypersensitivity to the drug. It should not be used in patients with preexisting myelosuppression resulting from prior drug therapy unless possible benefit warrants risk of further myelosuppression. Use with caution in patients with hepatic or renal impairment or preexisting cardiac disease.

Interactions

None reported.

Effects on diagnostic tests

Adverse effects of mitoxantrone may be reflected in abnormal hematologic or hepatic function tests. Serum uric acid levels may rise because of rapid lysis of tumor cells.

Adverse reactions

CNS: seizures, headache.
CV: *CHF, arrhythmia,* ECG changes, chest pain, tachycardia, hypotension, asymptomatic decreases in left ventricular ejection fraction.
DERM: alopecia, petechiae, ecchymosis, urticaria, rashes.

EENT: conjunctivitis.
GI: nausea, vomiting, diarrhea, abdominal pain, mucositis, stomatitis, bleeding.
GU: urinary tract infection, renal failure.
HEMA: thrombocytopenia, *leukopenia.*
Respiratory: cough, dyspnea, pneumonia.
Other: jaundice, sepsis, fungal infections, fever, phlebitis at injection site (rare), tissue necrosis after extravasation (rare).

Overdose and treatment

Accidental overdoses have occurred and have caused severe leukopenia with infection. Monitor hematologic parameters and treat symptomatically. Antimicrobial therapy may be necessary.

Special considerations

- Close and frequent monitoring of hematologic and chemical laboratory parameters, including serial CBC and liver function tests, with frequent patient observation is recommended.
- Safety of administration by routes other than I.V. has not been established. Do not use intrathecally.
- Hyperuricemia may result from rapid lysis of tumor cells. Monitor serum uric acid levels. Institute hypouricemic therapy before antileukemic therapy.
- Transient elevations of AST (formerly SGOT) and ALT (formerly SGPT) levels have occurred 4 to 24 days after mitoxantrone therapy.
- To prepare, dilute solutions to at least 50 ml with either 0.9% sodium chloride solution or dextrose 5% in water (D_5W). Inject slowly into tubing of a free-flowing I.V. solution of 0.9% sodium chloride solution or D_5W over not less than 3 minutes. Discard unused infusion solutions appropriately. Do not mix for infusion with heparin; a precipitate may form. Specific compatibility data are not available.
- If extravasation occurs, discontinue I.V. and restart in another vein. Mitoxantrone is a nonvesicant and the possibility of severe local reactions is minimal.
- Urine may appear blue-green for 24 hours after administration.

- Bluish discoloration of sclera may occur.

Information for the patient
- Tell patient urine may appear blue-green for 24 hours after administration and sclera may appear bluish.
- Advise patient to notify doctor promptly if signs and symptoms of myelosuppression (fever, sore throat, easy bruising, or excessive bleeding) develop.

pentostatin (2′-deoxycoformycin; DCF)
Nipent

Pregnancy risk category: D

How supplied

Powder for injection: 10-mg vial

Indications, route, and dosage

Alpha-interferon–refractory hairy-cell leukemia
Adults: 4 mg/m² I.V. every other week.

Pharmacodynamics

Pentostatin inhibits the enzyme adenosine deaminase (ADA), causing an increase in intracellular levels of deoxyadenosine triphosphate. This increase leads to cell damage and death. Because ADA is most active in cells of the lymphatic system (especially malignant T cells), pentostatin is useful in treating leukemias.

Pharmacokinetics

Absorption: Drug is given I.V.
Distribution: Plasma protein-binding is low (about 4%); distribution half-life is about 11 minutes.
Metabolism: Unknown.
Excretion: Over 90% of drug is excreted in urine. Clearance depends on renal function; mean terminal half-life is about 6 hours in patients with normal renal function and increases to 18 hours or more in patients with renal impairment (creatinine clearance below 50 ml/minute).

Contraindications and precautions

Pentostatin is contraindicated in patients with hypersensitivity to the drug. It should be used cautiously and only under supervision of a doctor qualified and experienced in the use of cancer chemotherapeutic drugs. Adverse reactions to pentostatin therapy are common.

Withhold or discontinue pentostatin in patients with evidence of CNS toxicity; also withhold the drug if the patient has a severe rash. Do not give to the patient who has an active infection; resume pentostatin therapy when infection clears. Avoid use in patients with renal damage (creatinine clearance of 60 ml/minute or less).

If the pretreatment level was over 500/mm^3, temporarily withhold the drug when the absolute neutrophil count falls below 200/mm^3. There are no recommendations regarding dosage adjustments in patients with anemia, neutropenia, or thrombocytopenia.

Interactions

Concomitant use with fludarabine increases the risk of severe or fatal pulmonary toxicity. Don't use together. Concomitant use with vidarabine increases the incidence or severity of adverse effects associated with either drug.

Effects on diagnostic tests

None reported.

Adverse reactions

CNS: headache, neurologic symptoms, anxiety, confusion, depression, dizziness, insomnia, nervousness, paresthesia, somnolence, abnormal thinking.
CV: *arrhythmias,* abnormal ECG, thrombophlebitis, hemorrhage.
DERM: ecchymosis, petechiae, rash, skin disorder, eczema, dry skin, herpes simplex, herpes zoster, maculopapular rash, vesiculobullous rash, pruritus, seborrhea, discoloration, sweating.
EENT: abnormal vision, conjunctivitis, ear pain, eye pain, epistaxis, pharyngitis, rhinitis, sinusitis.

GI: nausea, vomiting, anorexia, diarrhea, constipation, flatulence, stomatitis.

GU: GU disorder, hematuria, dysuria, increased BUN level, increased creatinine level.

HEMA: *myelosuppression*, leukopenia, anemia, thrombocytopenia, lymphadenopathy.

Hepatic: elevated liver function tests.

Metabolic: weight loss, peripheral edema, increased LDH levels.

Respiratory: cough, upper respiratory disorder, lung disorder, bronchitis, dyspnea, *lung edema, pneumonia.*

Other: fever, infection, fatigue, pain, *allergic reactions*, chills, sepsis, chest pain, abdominal pain, back pain, flulike syndrome, asthenia, malaise, myalgia, arthralgia.

Overdose and treatment

High dosage of pentostatin (20 to 50 mg/m² in divided doses over 5 days) has been associated with deaths from severe CNS, hepatic, pulmonary, and renal toxicity. No specific antidote is known. If overdosage occurs, treat symptoms and provide supportive care.

Special considerations

- Pentostatin should be used only in patients who have hairy-cell leukemia refractory to alpha-interferon; that is, for disease that progresses after a minimum of 3 months of treatment with alpha-interferon or does not respond after 6 months of therapy.
- Optimal duration of therapy is unknown. Current recommendations call for two additional courses of therapy after a complete response. If patient hasn't had a partial response after 6 months of therapy, discontinue drug. If patient has had only a partial response, continue drug for another 6 months or for two courses of therapy after a complete response.
- Store powder for injection in the refrigerator (36° to 46° F [2° to 8° C]). Reconstituted and diluted solutions should be used within 8 hours because solution contains no preservative.
- Follow appropriate guidelines for proper handling, administration, and disposal of chemotherapeutic drugs. Treat

all spills and waste products with 5% sodium hypochlorite solution. Wear protective clothing and polyethylene gloves.

• To prepare and administer: Add 5 ml sterile water for injection to the vial containing pentostatin powder for injection. Mix thoroughly to make a solution of 5 mg/ml. Administer drug by I.V. bolus injection, or dilute further in 25 or 50 ml of dextrose 5% in water (D$_5$W) or 0.9% sodium chloride solution and infuse over 20 to 30 minutes.

• Be sure patient is adequately hydrated before therapy. Administer 500 to 1,000 ml of D$_5$W in 0.45% sodium chloride solution. Give 500 ml of D$_5$W after drug is given.

• Before therapy, assess renal function with a serum creatinine or creatinine clearance assay; repeat determinations periodically. Perform baseline and periodic determinations of CBC. Bone marrow aspirates and biopsies may be required at 2- to 3-month intervals to assess response to treatment.

plicamycin (formerly mithramycin)
Mithracin

Pregnancy risk category: X

How supplied

Injection: 2.5-mg vials

Indications, route, and dosage

Indications and dosage may vary. Check current literature for recommended protocol.
Testicular cancer
Men: 25 to 30 mcg/kg I.V. daily over a period of 4 to 6 hours for up to 10 days (based on ideal body weight or actual weight, whichever is less).
Hypercalcemia
Adults: 15 to 25 mcg/kg I.V. daily over a period of 4 to 6 hours for 3 to 4 days. Repeat at intervals of 1 week as needed.

Pharmacodynamics

Plicamycin exerts its cytotoxic activity by intercalating between DNA base pairs and also binding to the outside of the

---

DNA molecule. The result is inhibition of DNA-dependent RNA synthesis.

The exact mechanism by which plicamycin lowers serum calcium levels is unknown. Plicamycin may block the hypercalcemic effect of vitamin D or may inhibit the effect of parathyroid hormone on osteoclasts, preventing osteolysis. Both mechanisms reduce serum calcium concentrations.

Pharmacokinetics

Absorption: Plicamycin must be administered I.V.
Distribution: Plicamycin distributes mainly into the Kupffer cells of the liver, into renal tubular cells, and along formed bone surfaces. The drug also crosses the blood-brain barrier and achieves appreciable concentrations in CSF.
Metabolism: The metabolic fate of plicamycin is unclear.
Excretion: Plicamycin is eliminated primarily through the kidneys.

Contraindications and precautions

Plicamycin is contraindicated in patients with impaired bone marrow function, thrombocytopenia, thrombocytopathy, coagulation disorders, or electrolyte imbalance because it may worsen the symptoms associated with these disorders.

Exercise caution in patients with hepatic and renal dysfunction and in those who have previously received abdominal or mediastinal radiation, because these patients may be more susceptible to the drug's toxic effects.

Interactions

None reported.

Effects on diagnostic tests

Because of drug-induced toxicity, plicamycin therapy may increase serum concentrations of alkaline phosphatase, AST (formerly SGOT), ALT (formerly SGPT), LDH, and bilirubin; it may also increase serum creatinine and BUN levels through nephrotoxicity.

Adverse reactions

CNS: severe headache, lethargy.
DERM: periorbital pallor, usually the day before toxic symptoms occur; facial flushing.
GI: nausea, vomiting, anorexia, diarrhea, stomatitis, metallic taste.
GU: proteinuria; increased BUN and serum creatinine levels.
HEMA: *bone marrow depression* (dose-limiting); *thrombocytopenia; bleeding syndrome,* from epistaxis to generalized hemorrhage; depression of clotting factors; *leukopenia.*
Metabolic: decreased serum calcium, potassium, and phosphorus levels.
Local: extravasation causes irritation and cellulitis.

Overdose and treatment

Clinical manifestations of overdose include myelosuppression, electrolyte imbalance, and coagulation disorders.

Treatment is usually supportive and includes transfusion of blood components and appropriate symptomatic therapy. Patient's renal and hepatic status should be closely monitored.

Special considerations

- To reconstitute drug, use 4.9 ml of sterile water to give a concentration of 0.5 mg/ml. Reconstitute drug immediately before administration, and discard any unused solution.
- Plicamycin may be further diluted with 0.9% sodium chloride solution or dextrose 5% in water (D₅W) to a volume of 1,000 ml and administered as an I.V. infusion over 4 to 6 hours.
- Plicamycin may be administered by I.V. push injection, but this method is discouraged because of the higher incidence and greater severity of GI toxicity. Nausea and vomiting are greatly diminished as the infusion rate is decreased.
- Infusions of plicamycin in 1,000 ml D₅W are stable for up to 24 hours.
- If the I.V. infiltrates, stop the infusion immediately and apply ice packs before restarting the I.V. in the other arm.

- To reduce nausea, give antiemetics before administering drug.
- Monitor LDH, AST, ALT, alkaline phosphatase, BUN, creatinine, potassium, calcium, and phosphorus levels.
- Monitor platelet count and prothrombin time before and during therapy.
- Check serum calcium levels. Monitor patient for tetany, carpopedal spasm, Chvostek's sign, and muscle cramps, because a precipitous drop in calcium levels is possible.
- Observe for signs of bleeding. Facial flushing may be an early indication of a patient developing a bleeding complication.
- Therapeutic effect in hypercalcemia may not be seen for 24 to 48 hours; may last 3 to 15 days.
- Avoid drug contact with skin or mucous membranes.
- Store lyophilized powder in refrigerator.

Information for the patient
- Tell patient to use salicylate-free medication for pain relief or fever reduction.
- Tell patient to avoid exposure to persons with infections.
- Patient should not receive immunizations during therapy and for several weeks after therapy. Members of the patient's household should not receive immunizations during the same period.

procarbazine hydrochloride
Matulane, Natulan
Pregnancy risk category: D

How supplied
Capsules: 50 mg

Indications, route, and dosage
Indications and dosage may vary. Check current literature for recommended protocol.

Hodgkin's disease, lymphomas, brain and lung cancers
Adults: 2 to 4 mg/kg/day P.O. in single or divided doses for the first week, followed by 4 to 6 mg/kg/day until response or toxicity occurs. Maintenance dosage is 1 to 2 mg/kg/day.
Children: 50 mg P.O. daily for first week, then 100 mg/m² until response or toxicity occurs. Maintenance dosage is 50 mg P.O. daily after bone marrow recovery.

Pharmacodynamics

The exact mechanism of procarbazine's cytotoxic activity is unknown. The drug appears to have several sites of action; the result is inhibition of DNA, RNA, and protein synthesis. Procarbazine has also been reported to damage DNA directly and to inhibit the mitotic S phase of cell division.

Pharmacokinetics

Absorption: Procarbazine is rapidly and completely absorbed after oral administration.
Distribution: Procarbazine distributes widely into body tissues, with the highest concentrations found in the liver, kidneys, intestinal wall, and skin. The drug crosses the blood-brain barrier.
Metabolism: Procarbazine is extensively metabolized in the liver. Some of the metabolites have cytotoxic activity.
Excretion: Procarbazine and its metabolites are excreted primarily in urine.

Contraindications and precautions

Procarbazine is contraindicated in patients with a history of hypersensitivity to the drug and in patients with poor bone marrow reserve because of potential for serious toxicity.

Procarbazine should be used cautiously in patients with hepatic or renal impairment because of potential for drug accumulation, in those with infections or leukopenia because of decreased immune response, and in those taking concurrent CNS depressants or MAO inhibitors because the drug has MAO-inhibiting activity. Also use cautiously in patients with thrombocytopenia or anemia.

Interactions

Concomitant use of procarbazine with alcohol can cause a disulfiram-like reaction. The mechanism of this interaction is poorly defined. Concomitant use with CNS depressants enhances CNS depression through an additive mechanism; concomitant use with sympathomimetics, tricyclic antidepressants, MAO inhibitors, or tyramine-rich foods can cause a hypertensive crisis, tremors, excitation, and cardiac palpitations through inhibition of MAO by procarbazine. Serum digoxin levels may be decreased. Concomitant use with meperidine may result in severe hypotension and death.

Effects on diagnostic tests

None reported.

Adverse reactions

CNS: paresthesias, myalgias, arthralgias, fatigue, lethargy, nervousness, depression, insomnia, nightmares, hallucinations, confusion.
DERM: dermatitis, pruritus, flushing, hyperpigmentation, photosensitivity.
EENT: retinal hemorrhage, nystagmus, photophobia, diplopia, papilledema, altered hearing.
GI: nausea, vomiting, anorexia, stomatitis, dry mouth, dysphagia, diarrhea, constipation.
GU: decreased spermatogenesis, infertility.
HEMA: *bone marrow depression* (dose-limiting), *pancytopenia, hemolysis,* bleeding tendency, *thrombocytopenia, leukopenia,* anemia.
Other: chills, fever, pneumonitis, hypotension, reversible alopecia, pleural effusion.
   Note: Drug should be discontinued if the following occur: bleeding or bleeding tendencies, stomatitis, diarrhea, paresthesias, neuropathies, confusion, or hypersensitivity.

Overdose and treatment

Clinical manifestations of overdose include myalgia, arthralgia, fever, weakness, dermatitis, alopecia, paresthesias, hallucinations, tremors, seizure, coma, myelosuppression, nausea, and vomiting.

Treatment is usually supportive and includes transfusion of blood components, antiemetics, antipyretics, and appropriate antianxiety agents.

Special considerations

• Nausea and vomiting may be decreased if procarbazine is taken at bedtime and in divided doses.
• Observe for signs of bleeding.
• Store capsules in dry environment.

Information for the patient

• Emphasize importance of continuing medication despite nausea and vomiting.
• Advise patient to call immediately if vomiting occurs shortly after taking dose.
• Warn patient that drowsiness may occur, so patient should avoid hazardous activities that require alertness until drug's effect is established.
• Warn patient not to drink alcoholic beverages while taking this drug.
• Instruct patient to stop medication and call immediately if disulfiram-like reaction (chest pains, rapid or irregular heartbeat, severe headache, stiff neck) occurs.
• Tell patient to avoid exposure to persons with infections.
• Warn patient to avoid prolonged exposure to the sun because photosensitivity occurs during therapy.
• Tell patient to report a sore throat or fever or any unusual bruising or bleeding.

streptozocin
Zanosar

Pregnancy risk category: C

How supplied

Injection: 1-g vials

Indications, route, and dosage

Indications and dosage may vary. Check current literature for recommended protocol.

Metastatic islet cell carcinoma of the pancreas, colon cancer, exocrine pancreatic tumors, carcinoid tumors

Adults and children: 500 mg/m² I.V. for 5 consecutive days q 4 to 6 weeks until maximum benefit or toxicity is observed. Alternatively, 1,000 mg/m² at weekly intervals for the first 2 weeks, increased to a maximum single dose of 1,500 mg/m². Usual course of therapy is 4 to 6 weeks.

Pharmacodynamics

Streptozocin exerts its cytotoxic activity by selectively inhibiting DNA synthesis. The drug also causes cross-linking of DNA strands through an alkylation mechanism.

Pharmacokinetics

Absorption: Streptozocin is not active orally and must be given I.V.

Distribution: Streptozocin and its metabolites distribute mainly into the liver, kidneys, intestines, and pancreas. The drug has not been shown to cross the blood-brain barrier; however, its metabolites achieve concentrations in CSF equivalent to the concentration in the plasma.

Metabolism: Streptozocin is extensively metabolized in the liver and kidneys.

Excretion: The elimination of streptozocin from the plasma is biphasic, with an initial half-life of 5 minutes and a terminal phase half-life of 35 to 40 minutes. The plasma half-life of the metabolites is longer than that of the parent drug. The drug and its metabolites are excreted primarily in urine. A small amount of a dose may also be excreted in expired air.

Contraindications and precautions

No contraindications have been reported for streptozocin.

Streptozocin should be used cautiously in patients with renal or hepatic dysfunction or hematologic compromise. Dosage adjustments are necessary.

Interactions

When used concomitantly, other nephrotoxic drugs may potentiate the nephrotoxicity caused by streptozocin. Concomitant use with doxorubicin prolongs the elimination half-life of doxorubicin and requires reduced dosage of doxorubicin.

Concurrent use with phenytoin may decrease the effects of streptozocin on the pancreas.

Effects on diagnostic tests

Streptozocin therapy may decrease serum albumin and increase liver function test values; these increases are a sign of hepatotoxicity. BUN and serum creatinine levels may be increased, indicating nephrotoxicity. The drug may decrease blood glucose levels because of a sudden release of insulin.

Adverse reactions

CNS: lethargy, confusion.
GI: nausea and vomiting (dose-limiting), diarrhea.
GU: renal toxicity (evidenced by azotemia, glycosuria, and renal tubular acidosis), mild proteinuria.
HEMA: *leukopenia, thrombocytopenia,* anemia.
Hepatic: elevated liver enzyme levels, liver dysfunction.
Metabolic: hyperglycemia, hypoglycemia.
Local: sloughing, severe irritation if extravasation occurs.

Overdose and treatment

Clinical manifestations of overdose include myelosuppression, nausea, and vomiting.

Treatment is usually supportive and includes transfusion of blood components and administration of antiemetics.

Special considerations

- To reconstitute streptozocin, use 9.5 ml of 0.9% sodium chloride injection to yield a concentration of 100 mg/ml.
- If possible, use streptozocin within 12 hours of reconstitution. The reconstituted solution is a golden color that changes to dark brown on decomposition.
- The product contains no preservatives and is not intended for use as a multiple-dose vial.
- Streptozocin may be administered by rapid I.V. push.
- Streptozocin may be further diluted in 10 to 200 ml of dextrose 5% in water to infuse over 10 to 15 minutes. It can also be infused over 6 hours.
- Wear gloves during preparation or administration to protect the skin from contact. If contact occurs, wash solution

---

off immediately with soap and water. Follow the recommended procedures for the safe preparation, administration, and disposal of chemotherapeutic drugs.

- Extravasation may cause ulceration and tissue necrosis.
- Phenytoin may be administered concomitantly to protect pancreatic beta cells from cytotoxicity.
- Keep dextrose 50% at bedside because of risk of hypoglycemia from sudden release of insulin.
- Nausea and vomiting occur in almost all patients within 1 to 4 hours. Make sure patient is being treated with an antiemetic.
- Mild proteinuria is one of the first signs of renal toxicity and may require dosage reduction.
- Urine should be tested regularly for protein and glucose.
- Monitor CBC and liver function studies at least weekly.
- Renal toxicity resulting from streptozocin therapy is dose related and cumulative. Monitor renal function before and after each course of therapy. Obtain urinalysis, BUN levels, and creatinine clearance before therapy and at least weekly during drug administration. Continue weekly monitoring for 4 weeks after each course.

Information for the patient

- Encourage adequate fluid intake to increase urine output and reduce potential for renal toxicity.
- Remind diabetic patients that intensive monitoring of blood glucose levels is necessary.
- Tell patient to report any symptoms of anemia, infection, or bleeding immediately.

Antimetabolites

cytarabine   mercaptopurine

floxuridine   methotrexate

fludarabine phosphate   thioguanine

fluorouracil   trimetrexate glucuronate

Antimetabolites compete with naturally occurring substrates to disrupt cellular metabolism. Most are structural analogs of normally occurring metabolites and can be divided into three subcategories: purine analogs, pyrimidine analogs, and folic acid analogs. Most of these agents interrupt cell reproduction at a specific phase of the cell cycle and are most effective against tumors with a high growth fraction (that is, high numbers or high proportion of cells dividing at any one time).

Pharmacology

The mechanism of action of each antimetabolite subcategory differs according to the function with which the drug interferes. The purine analogs are incorporated into DNA and RNA, interfering with nucleic acid synthesis (by miscoding) and replication. They may also inhibit the synthesis of purine bases through pseudofeedback mechanisms. Pyrimidine analogs inhibit enzymes active in biosynthesis of uridine and thymine. Folic acid antagonists prevent conversion of dehydrofolate to tetrahydrofolate by inhibiting the enzyme dihydrofolic acid reductase.

Antimetabolites may slow the entry of some cells into the S phase, thus sparing these cells from the drug's cytotoxic effects. Because most antimetabolites act in the S phase, this slowing effect may limit their cytotoxicity.

Clinical indications and actions

Antimetabolites are useful alone or in combination with other types of antineoplastic agents for treating various tumors. For specific uses, see the individual drug entries in this chapter.

Overview of adverse reactions

The most frequent adverse reactions to antimetabolites include nausea, vomiting, diarrhea, fever, chills, possible alopecia, flank or joint pain, redness or pain at injection site, anxiety, bone marrow depression, leukopenia, and swelling of feet or lower legs.

Special considerations

- Follow all established procedures for the safe and proper handling, administration, and disposal of chemotherapeutic drugs.
- Monitor vital signs and patency of catheter or I.V. line throughout administration.
- Treat extravasations promptly.
- Attempt to alleviate or reduce anxiety in patient and family before treatment.
- Monitor BUN; hematocrit; platelet count and total and differential WBC count; ALT (formerly SGPT), AST (formerly SGOT), LDH, serum bilirubin, serum creatinine, and uric acid levels; and other test results as required.
- Immunizations should be avoided if possible.

Information for the patient

- Instruct patient in proper oral hygiene, including caution when using toothbrush, dental floss, and toothpicks. Chemotherapy can increase incidence of microbial infection, delayed healing, and bleeding gums.
- Tell patient to complete dental work before initiation of therapy whenever possible, or to delay it until blood counts are normal.

- Warn patient that he may bruise easily because of drug's effect on platelet counts.
- Warn patient to avoid close contact with persons who have taken oral poliovirus vaccine and to avoid exposure to persons with bacterial or viral infection, because chemotherapy may increase susceptibility to infection. Instruct him to report signs of infection immediately.
- Tell patient to report immediately any redness, pain, or swelling at the injection site. Local tissue injury and scarring may result from tissue infiltration at the infusion site.

cytarabine (ara-C, cytosine arabinoside)
Cytosar-U

Pregnancy risk category: D

How supplied

Injection: 100-mg, 500-mg, 1-g, 2-g vials

Indications, route, and dosage

Indications and dosage may vary. Check literature for recommended protocol.

Acute myelocytic and other acute leukemias

Adults and children: 100 to 200 mg/m^2 or 3 mg/kg daily by continuous I.V. infusion or rapid I.V. injection in divided doses for 5 days at 2-week intervals for remission induction, or 30 mg/m^2 intrathecally (range: 5 to 75 mg/m^2) q 4 days until CSF findings are normal. Doses up to 3 g/m^2 q 12 hours for 12 doses have been given by continuous infusion for refractory acute leukemias.

Pharmacodynamics

Cytarabine requires conversion to its active metabolite within the cell. This metabolite acts as a competitive inhibitor of the enzyme DNA polymerase, disrupting the normal synthesis of DNA.

Pharmacokinetics

Absorption: Cytarabine is poorly absorbed (less than 20%) across the GI tract because of rapid deactivation in the gut lumen. After I.M. or S.C. administration, peak plasma levels are lower than after I.V. administration.

Distribution: Cytarabine rapidly distributes widely through the body. Approximately 13% of the drug is bound to plasma proteins. The drug penetrates the blood-brain barrier only slightly after a single I.V. dose; however, when cytarabine is administered by continuous I.V. infusion, CSF levels elevate and may reach 40% to 60% of plasma concentration.

Metabolism: Cytarabine is metabolized primarily in the liver but also in the kidneys, GI mucosa, and granulocytes.

Excretion: Cytarabine elimination is biphasic, with an initial half-life of about 8 minutes and a terminal phase half-life of about 1 to 3 hours. Cytarabine and its metabolites are excreted in urine. Less than 10% of a dose is excreted as unchanged drug in urine.

Contraindications and precautions

Cytarabine is contraindicated in patients with a history of hypersensitivity to the drug. Cytarabine is a highly toxic drug. Therapeutic response is usually accompanied by toxicity. Drug-induced myelosuppression may make patients susceptible to hemorrhagic complications or to viral, bacterial, or fungal infections.

Interactions

When used concomitantly with methotrexate, cytarabine decreases the cellular uptake of methotrexate, reducing its effectiveness. Temporary damage to GI mucosa produced by cytarabine may impair oral absorption of digoxin.

Effects on diagnostic tests

Cytarabine therapy may increase blood and urine levels of uric acid. It may also increase serum alkaline phosphatase, AST (formerly SGOT), and bilirubin concentrations, which are signs of drug-induced hepatotoxicity.

---

*Canada only   †Off-label use   Italicized adverse reactions are life-threatening.

Adverse reactions

CNS: neurotoxicity; cerebellar dysfunction, neuritis and peripheral neuropathy (with high doses).
DERM: rash, alopecia.
EENT: keratitis.
GI: nausea; vomiting; diarrhea; dysphagia; reddened area at juncture of lips, followed by sore mouth, oral ulcers in 5 to 10 days; projectile vomiting (with high dose given rapid I.V.).
HEMA: *leukopenia* (nadir 7 to 9 days after drug discontinued), anemia, *thrombocytopenia*, reticulocytopenia (platelet nadir occurring on day 10), *megaloblastosis, bone marrow depression* (dose-limiting). *Note:* Drug should be discontinued if the polymorphonuclear granulocyte count falls below 1,000/mm³ or if the platelet count falls below 50,000/mm³ during maintenance therapy (not during remission induction therapy).
Hepatic: hepatotoxicity (usually mild and reversible).
Metabolic: hyperuricemia.
Other: flulike syndrome.

Overdose and treatment

Clinical manifestations of overdose include myelosuppression, nausea, vomiting, and megaloblastosis.

Treatment is usually supportive and includes transfusion of blood components and administration of antiemetics.

Special considerations

- To reconstitute for I.V. administration, add 5 ml bacteriostatic water for injection to the 100-mg vial to give a concentration of 20 mg/ml; add 10 ml bacteriostatic water for injection to the 500-mg vial to give a concentration of 50 mg/ml.
- Cytarabine may be further diluted with dextrose 5% in water or 0.9% sodium chloride solution for continuous I.V. infusion.
- For intrathecal injection, dilute the drug in 5 to 15 ml of lactated Ringer's solution, Elliot's B solution, or 0.9% sodium chloride solution with no preservative, and administer after withdrawing an equivalent volume of CSF.

- Do not reconstitute the drug with bacteriostatic diluent for intrathecal administration because benzyl alcohol, the preservative, has been associated with a higher incidence of neurotoxicity.
- Reconstituted solutions are stable for 48 hours at room temperature. Infusion solutions up to a concentration of 5 mg/ml are stable for 7 days at room temperature. Discard cloudy reconstituted solution.
- Dose modification may be required in patients with thrombocytopenia, leukopenia, renal or hepatic disease, and after other chemotherapy or radiation therapy.
- Watch for signs of infection (cough, fever, sore throat). Monitor CBC.
- Provide excellent mouth care to help prevent adverse oral reactions.
- Nausea and vomiting are more frequent when large doses are administered rapidly by I.V. push. These reactions are less frequent with infusion. To reduce nausea, give anti-emetic before administering.
- Monitor intake and output carefully. Maintain high fluid intake and give allopurinol, if ordered, to avoid urate nephropathy in remission induction therapy. Monitor uric acid levels.
- Monitor hepatic function.
- Monitor patients receiving high doses for cerebellar dysfunction.
- Ensure that patient receives steroid eyedrops (dexamethasone) to prevent drug-induced keratitis.
- Avoid any I.M. injections in patients with severely depressed platelet count to prevent bleeding.
- Pyridoxine supplements may be administered to prevent neuropathies; reportedly, however, prophylactic use of pyridoxine does not prevent cytarabine neurotoxicity.

Information for the patient
- Encourage adequate fluid intake to increase urine output and facilitate uric acid excretion.
- Tell the patient to notify the doctor immediately if sore throat, fever, or unusual bruising or bleeding occurs.
- Advise patient to avoid exposure to persons with infections.

- Provide detailed mouth care instructions. Stress to the patient and caregiver that diligent mouth care can prevent oral adverse reactions.

floxuridine
FUDR

Pregnancy risk category: C

How supplied

Injection: 500-mg vials

Indications, route, and dosage

Indications and dosage may vary. Check current literature for recommended protocol.
Brain, breast, head, neck, liver, gallbladder, and bile duct cancers
Adults: 0.1 to 0.6 mg/kg daily by intra-arterial infusion, or 0.4 to 0.6 mg/kg daily into hepatic artery.

Pharmacodynamics

Floxuridine exerts its cytotoxic activity after conversion to its active form by competitively inhibiting the enzyme thymidylate synthetase; this halts DNA synthesis and leads to cell death.

Pharmacokinetics

Absorption: Floxuridine must be administered I.V. because of poor oral absorption.
Distribution: Floxuridine crosses the blood-brain barrier to a limited extent.
Metabolism: Floxuridine is metabolized to fluorouracil in the liver after intra-arterial infusions and rapid I.V. injections.
Excretion: About 60% of a dose of floxuridine is excreted through the lungs as carbon dioxide. A small amount is excreted by the kidneys as unchanged drug and metabolites.

Contraindications and precautions

Floxuridine is a highly toxic drug. Therapeutic response is usually accompanied by toxicity.

Floxuridine is contraindicated in patients with poor nutritional status, depressed bone marrow function, or serious infections because these patients are at high risk for serious drug-related toxicity. Drug-induced hematologic toxicity may leave patients susceptible to severe hemorrhagic complications.

Use cautiously in patients who are receiving alkylating agents or high-dose pelvic irradiation therapy. If myocardial ischemia or intractable nausea and vomiting occurs, discontinue the drug immediately.

Interactions

None significant.

Effects on diagnostic tests

Floxuridine therapy may increase serum concentrations of ALT (formerly SGPT), alkaline phosphatase, AST (formerly SGOT), bilirubin, and LDH; these increases indicate drug-induced hepatotoxicity.

Adverse reactions

CNS: cerebellar ataxia, vertigo, nystagmus, *seizures*, depression, hemiplegia, hiccups, lethargy.
DERM: erythema, dermatitis, pruritus, rash.
EENT: blurred vision.
GI: stomatitis, cramps, nausea, vomiting, diarrhea, GI bleeding, enteritis.
HEMA: *bone marrow depression* (dose-limiting), *leukopenia*, anemia, *thrombocytopenia*.
Hepatic: cholangitis, jaundice, elevated liver enzyme levels.
Note: Drug should be discontinued if stomatitis, GI bleeding, esophagopharyngitis, or thromboembolic events occur; if the WBC count falls below 3,500/mm^3; or if the platelet count falls below 100,000/mm^3.

Overdose and treatment

Clinical manifestations of floxuridine overdose include myelosuppression, diarrhea, alopecia, dermatitis, and hyperpigmentation.

Treatment is usually supportive and includes transfusion of blood components and administration of antidiarrheal agents.

Special considerations

- To reconstitute, add 5 ml sterile water for injection to give a concentration of 100 mg/ml.
- Dilute to appropriate volume for infusion device with dextrose 5% in water or 0.9% sodium chloride solution.
- Administration by infusion pump maintains a continuous, uniform rate. Reconstituted floxuridine solutions are stable for 14 days when refrigerated.
- Observe arterial perfused area. Check line for bleeding, blockage, displacement, or leakage.
- Floxuridine is often administered by hepatic arterial infusion to treat hepatic metastases.
- Severe cardiac, hematologic, skin, or GI adverse reactions require discontinuing floxuridine therapy.
- Provide excellent mouth care to help prevent oral adverse reactions.
- Monitor intake and output, CBC, and renal and hepatic function.
- Therapeutic effect may be delayed 1 to 6 weeks. Make sure patient is aware of time required for improvement.
- To prevent bleeding, avoid I.M. injections of any drugs in patients with thrombocytopenia.
- Floxuridine may be given concurrently with doxorubicin in the same infusion.

Information for the patient
- Advise patient to report nausea, vomiting, stomach pain, or any unusual bruising or bleeding.
- Provide detailed mouth care instructions. Stress to the patient and caregiver that diligent mouth care can prevent adverse oral reactions.

fludarabine phosphate
Fludara

Pregnancy risk category: D

How supplied

Injection: 50 mg as lyophilized powder

Indications, route, and dosage

B-cell chronic lymphocytic leukemia (CLL) in patients who have not responded or have responded inadequately to at least one standard alkylating agent regimen
Adults: Usually, 25 mg/m² I.V. over 30 minutes for 5 consecutive days q 28 days. Therapy based on patient response and tolerance.

Pharmacodynamics

After rapid conversion of fludarabine to its active metabolite, the metabolite appears to inhibit DNA synthesis by inhibiting DNA polymerase alpha, ribonucleotide reductase, and DNA primase. The exact mechanism of action is not fully established.

Pharmacokinetics

Absorption: Fludarabine is administered I.V.
Metabolism: Fludarabine is rapidly dephosphorylated and then phosphorylated intracellularly to its active metabolite.
Distribution: Unknown.
Excretion: 23% of a dose is excreted in urine as unchanged active metabolite.

Contraindications and precautions

Fludarabine is a highly toxic drug. Therapeutic response is usually accompanied by toxicity. Drug-induced myelosuppression may leave patients susceptible to hemorrhagic complications or to viral, bacterial, or fungal infections. Potentially severe or fatal neurotoxicity can occur with high doses.

Fludarabine is contraindicated in patients with hypersensitivity to the drug or its components. Use cautiously in

---

patients with renal insufficiency, hematologic impairment, or myelosuppression.

Interactions

Concomitant use with other myelosuppressive agents may cause additive toxicity.

Effects on diagnostic tests

None reported.

Adverse reactions

CNS: fatigue, malaise, weakness, paresthesia, headache, sleep disorder, depression, cerebellar syndrome, agitation, confusion, peripheral neuropathy.
CV: edema, angina, phlebitis, arrhythmias, *CHF*, deep venous thrombosis, transient ischemic attack, aneurysm, *CVA*, hemorrhage.
DERM: rash, pruritus, seborrhea.
EENT: visual disturbances, hearing loss, sinusitis, epistaxis.
GI: nausea, vomiting, diarrhea, constipation, anorexia, stomatitis, GI bleeding, esophagitis, mucositis.
GU: dysuria, urinary infection, urinary hesitancy, proteinuria, hematuria, *renal failure*.
HEMA: thrombocytopenia, neutropenia, anemia.
Respiratory: cough, pneumonia, dyspnea, pharyngitis, allergic pneumonitis, hemoptysis, bronchitis.
Other: fever, chills, infection, pain, myalgia, tumor lysis syndrome, alopecia, *anaphylaxis*, diaphoresis, hyperglycemia, dehydration, *liver failure*, cholelithiasis.

Overdose and treatment

Irreversible CNS toxicity characterized by delayed blindness, coma, and death is associated with high doses. Severe thrombocytopenia and neutropenia secondary to bone marrow suppression also occur.

No specific antidote exists, and treatment consists of discontinuing therapy and taking supportive measures.

Special considerations

- Fludarabine should be administered under the supervision of a doctor experienced in antineoplastic therapy.
- Careful hematologic monitoring is required, especially of neutrophil and platelet counts.
- Tumor lysis syndrome (hyperuricemia, hyperphosphatemia, hypocalcemia, metabolic acidosis, hyperkalemia, hematuria, urate crystalluria, and renal failure) has occurred in CLL patients with large tumors.
- Severe neurologic effects are seen when high doses are used to treat acute leukemia.
- Advanced age, renal insufficiency, and bone marrow impairment may predispose patient to severe toxicity; toxic effects are dose-dependent.
- Optimal duration of therapy has not been established; three additional cycles after achieving maximal response are recommended before discontinuing drug.
- To prepare fludarabine, add 2 ml of sterile water for injection to the solid cake of the drug. Dissolution should occur within 15 seconds; each milliliter will contain 25 mg of drug, 25 mg of mannitol, and sodium hydroxide. Use within 8 hours of reconstitution. Dilute in 100 ml of dextrose 5% in water or 0.9% sodium chloride solution and infuse over 30 minutes.
- Follow the facility's protocol and guidelines for proper handling and disposal of chemotherapeutic drugs.
- Store drug in refrigerator at 35.6° to 46.4° F (2° to 8° C).
- Fludarabine is used investigationally in the treatment of non-Hodgkin's lymphoma, macroglobulinemic lymphoma, prolymphocytic leukemia or prolymphocytoid variant of CLL, mycosis fungoides, hairy-cell leukemia, and Hodgkin's disease.

Information for the patient
- Tell patient to avoid persons with infection during therapy.
- Remind patient that he should report adverse reactions promptly.

Geriatric use
Advanced age may increase toxicity potential.

---

fluorouracil (5-FU)
Adrucil, Efudex, Fluroplex
Pregnancy risk category: D

How supplied

Injection: 50 mg/ml in 10-ml, 20-ml vials; 1,000 mg/20-ml vials
Cream: 1%, 5%
Topical solution: 1%, 2%, 5%

Indications, route, and dosage

Indications and dosage may vary. Check current literature for recommended protocol.
Colon, rectal, breast, ovarian, cervical, gastric, esophageal, bladder, liver, pancreatic, and unknown primary cancers
Adults and children: 7 to 12 mg/kg I.V. for 4 days, then (after 3 days) 7 to 10 mg/kg q 3 to 4 days for 2 weeks. Alternatively, 12 mg/kg I.V. for 5 days, followed (after 1 day) by 6 mg/kg I.V. every other day for 4 or 5 doses, for a total course of 2 weeks. Maintenance infusion is 7 to 12 mg/kg I.V. q 7 to 10 days or 300 to 500 mg/m^2 q 4 to 5 days, repeated monthly. Do not exceed 800 mg/day (400 mg/day in severely ill patients).
Actinic or solar keratoses
Adults: Sufficient cream or lotion to cover lesions b.i.d. Usually, 1% preparations are used on head, neck, and chest; 2% and 5% on hands.
Superficial basal cell carcinomas
Adults: 5% solution or cream in a sufficient amount to cover lesion b.i.d.

Pharmacodynamics

Fluorouracil exerts its cytotoxic effect by acting as an antimetabolite, competing for an enzyme that is important in the synthesis of thymidine, an essential substrate for DNA synthesis. Therefore, DNA synthesis is inhibited. The drug also inhibits RNA synthesis to a lesser extent.

Pharmacokinetics

Absorption: Because fluorouracil is absorbed poorly after oral administration, it is given parenterally.

Distribution: Fluorouracil distributes widely into all areas of body water and tissues, including tumors, bone marrow, liver, and intestinal mucosa. Fluorouracil crosses the blood-brain barrier to a significant extent.

Metabolism: A small amount of fluorouracil is converted in the tissues to the active metabolite, with most of the drug degraded in the liver.

Excretion: Metabolites of fluorouracil are primarily excreted through the lungs as carbon dioxide. A small portion of a dose is excreted in urine as unchanged drug.

Contraindications and precautions

Fluorouracil is a toxic drug. Drug-induced myelosuppression may leave patients susceptible to hemorrhagic complications or to viral, bacterial, or fungal infections.

Fluorouracil is contraindicated in patients with poor nutritional status, depressed bone marrow function, or serious infections, or in those who have recently undergone major surgery, because of the increased potential for toxicity; it is contraindicated in pregnant patients because the drug may be fetotoxic.

Interactions

When used concomitantly, leucovorin calcium given as a continuous infusion causes increased binding of fluorouracil to substrate, increased fluorouracil cell uptake, and increased inhibition of thymidine synthetase. Significance is unknown.

Effects on diagnostic tests

Fluorouracil may decrease plasma albumin concentration because of drug-induced protein malabsorption.

Adverse reactions

CNS: acute cerebellar syndrome, drowsiness, euphoria.
CV: mild angina, ECG changes.

DERM: maculopapular rash, dryness, erythema, hyperpigmentation (especially in blacks), nail changes, pigmented palmar creases, pruritus, suppuration, burning, swelling, scarring.

GI: anorexia, proctitis, paralytic ileus, stomatitis, diarrhea (GI ulcer may precede leukopenia), nausea, vomiting, GI toxicity (dose-limiting).

HEMA: *bone marrow depression* (dose-limiting), *leukopenia* (nadir in 7 to 14 days), anemia, thrombocytopenia.

Other: photosensitivity, lacrimation, reversible alopecia, weakness, malaise.

Note: Drug should be discontinued if intractable vomiting, stomatitis, diarrhea, GI ulceration, or GI bleeding occurs; if the WBC count falls below 3,000/mm³; or if the platelet count falls below 100,000/mm³.

Overdose and treatment

Clinical manifestations of overdose include myelosuppression, diarrhea, alopecia, dermatitis, hyperpigmentation, nausea, and vomiting.

Treatment is usually supportive and includes transfusion of blood components and administration of antiemetics and antidiarrheals.

Special considerations

- To reconstitute fluorouracil, withdraw the solution through a 5-micron filter and add to vial.
- Fluorouracil may be administered I.V. push over 1 to 2 minutes.
- Fluorouracil may be further diluted in dextrose 5% in water or 0.9% sodium chloride solution for infusions up to 24 hours in duration.
- Use plastic I.V. containers for administering continuous infusions. Solution is more stable in plastic I.V. bags than in glass bottles.
- Do not use cloudy solution. If crystals form, redissolve by warming at 140° F (60° C). Allow solution to cool to body temperature before using.
- Use new vein site for each dose.
- To decrease nausea, give antiemetic before administering.

- If extravasation occurs, treat as a chemical phlebitis with warm compresses.
- Do not refrigerate fluorouracil.
- Fluorouracil can be diluted in 120 ml of a 0.2 M sodium bicarbonate solution and administered orally.
- General photosensitivity occurs for 2 to 3 months after a dose.
- Ingestion and systemic absorption may cause leukopenia, thrombocytopenia, stomatitis, diarrhea or GI ulceration, bleeding, and hemorrhage. A topical local anesthetic may be used to soothe mouth lesions. Encourage frequent mouth care.
- Monitor intake and output, CBC, and renal and hepatic function.
- Avoid I.M. injections in patients with low platelet counts.
- Don two pairs of high-grade, extra thick latex gloves to apply topical drug. Wash hands immediately after handling medication. Avoid occlusive dressings because they may increase the incidence of inflammatory reactions in normal skin surrounding affected areas.
- Apply topical solution with caution near eyes, nose, and mouth.
- Topical application to larger ulcerated areas may cause systemic toxicity.
- For superficial basal cell carcinoma confirmed by biopsy, use 5% strength. Apply 1% concentration on the face. Reserve higher concentrations for thicker-skinned areas or resistant lesions.
- Do not continue to treat lesions resistant to fluorouracil; a biopsy of these lesions should be performed.

Information for the patient
- Warn patient to avoid strong sunlight or ultraviolet light because it will intensify the skin reaction. Encourage use of sunscreens.
- Tell patient to avoid exposure to persons with infections.
- Reassure patient that hair should grow back after treatment is discontinued.
- Provide detailed mouth care instructions.
- Tell patient to apply topical fluorouracil with gloves and to wash hands thoroughly after application.

• Warn patient that treated area may be unsightly during therapy and for several weeks after therapy is discontinued. Complete healing may not occur until 1 or 2 months after treatment is discontinued.

mercaptopurine (6-MP)
Purinethol

Pregnancy risk category: D

How supplied

Tablets (scored): 50 mg

Indications, route, and dosage

Indications and dosage may vary. Check current literature for recommended protocol.
Acute lymphoblastic leukemia (in children), acute myeloblastic leukemia, chronic myelocytic leukemia
Adults: 2.5 mg/kg or 80 to 100 mg/m^2 P.O. daily as a single dose, up to 5 mg/kg daily. Maintenance dosage is 1.5 to 2.5 mg/kg P.O. daily.
Children age 5 and over: 1.5 mg/kg or 75 mg/m^2 P.O. daily. Maintenance dosage is 1.5 to 2.5 mg/kg P.O. daily.

Pharmacodynamics

Mercaptopurine is converted intracellularly to its active form, which exerts its cytotoxic antimetabolic effects by competing for an enzyme required for purine synthesis. This results in inhibition of DNA and RNA synthesis. Cross-resistance exists between mercaptopurine and thioguanine.

Pharmacokinetics

Absorption: Mercaptopurine absorption after an oral dose is incomplete and variable; approximately 50% of a dose is absorbed. Peak serum levels occur 2 hours after a dose.
Distribution: Mercaptopurine distributes widely into total body water. The drug crosses the blood-brain barrier, but the CSF concentration is too low for treatment of meningeal leukemias.

Metabolism: Mercaptopurine is extensively metabolized in the liver. The drug appears to undergo extensive first-pass metabolism, contributing to its low bioavailability.

Excretion: Mercaptopurine and its metabolites are excreted in urine.

Contraindications and precautions

Mercaptopurine is a highly toxic drug. Therapeutic response is usually accompanied by toxicity. Drug-induced myelosuppression may leave patients susceptible to hemorrhagic complications or to viral, bacterial, or fungal infections.

Mercaptopurine is contraindicated in patients whose disease has shown resistance to therapy with this drug. Complete cross-resistance usually exists between mercaptopurine and thioguanine.

Bone marrow suppression, resulting in anemia, leukopenia, or thrombocytopenia, is usually the most consistent dose-related toxicity.

The incidence of hepatotoxicity increases when doses exceed 2.5 mg/kg/day. Clinical jaundice usually occurs early in treatment, but there have been reports of patients taking the drug for 8 years before jaundice develops.

Interactions

When used concomitantly, allopurinol (at doses of 300 to 600 mg/day) increases the toxic effects of mercaptopurine, especially myelosuppression. This is due to the inhibition of mercaptopurine metabolism by allopurinol. Reduce dosage of mercaptopurine to 25% to 30% when administering concomitantly with allopurinol.

Concomitant use of warfarin with mercaptopurine decreases the anticoagulant activity of warfarin. The mechanism of this interaction is unknown.

Mercaptopurine should be used cautiously with other hepatotoxic drugs because of the increased potential for hepatotoxicity.

Effects on diagnostic tests

Mercaptopurine therapy may cause falsely elevated serum glucose and uric acid values when sequential multiple analyzer is used.

Adverse reactions

DERM: hyperpigmentation, rash.

GI: nausea, vomiting, and anorexia in 25% of patients; painful oral ulcers.

HEMA: *bone marrow depression* (dose-limiting), decreased RBC count, *leukopenia, thrombocytopenia,* anemia (all may persist several days after drug therapy is discontinued).

Hepatic: jaundice, *hepatic necrosis.*

Metabolic: hyperuricemia.

Other: fever, headache.

Note: Drug should be discontinued if signs of bone marrow toxicity or toxic hepatitis occur.

Overdose and treatment

Clinical manifestations of overdose include myelosuppression, nausea, vomiting, and hepatic necrosis.

Treatment is usually supportive and includes transfusion of blood components and administration of antiemetics. Mercaptopurine is dialyzable.

Special considerations

- Adverse GI reactions occur less frequently in children than in adults.
- Store tablets at room temperature and protect from light.
- Dose modifications may be required following chemotherapy or radiation therapy, in patients with depressed neutrophil or platelet count, and in patients with impaired hepatic or renal function.
- Monitor intake and output. Push fluids (3 liters daily).
- Drug is sometimes called 6-mercaptopurine or 6-MP.
- Monitor hepatic function and hematologic values weekly during therapy. Watch for precipitous fall in blood counts.
- Monitor serum uric acid levels. If allopurinol is necessary, use very cautiously.
- Observe for signs of bleeding and infection.
- Hepatic dysfunction is reversible when drug is discontinued. Watch for jaundice, clay-colored stools, and frothy dark urine. Drug should be stopped if hepatic tenderness occurs.

---

*Canada only   †Off-label use   Italicized adverse reactions are life-threatening.

- Avoid all I.M. injections when platelet count is below 100,000/mm³.

Information for the patient
- Warn patient that improvement may take 2 to 4 weeks or longer.
- Tell patient to continue medication despite nausea and vomiting.
- Tell patient to report vomiting that occurs shortly after taking a dose.
- Warn patient to avoid alcoholic beverages while taking mercaptopurine.
- Urge patient to ensure adequate fluid intake, to increase urine output and facilitate uric acid excretion.
- Tell patient to avoid exposure to persons with infections.

methotrexate, methotrexate sodium
Folex, Mexate

Pregnancy risk category: D

How supplied

Tablets (scored): 2.5 mg
Injection: 20-mg, 25-mg, 50-mg, 100-mg, 250-mg, 1-g vials, ly-ophilized powder, preservative-free; 25-mg/ml vials, preservative-free solution; 2.5-mg/ml, 25-mg/ml vials, lyophilized powder, preserved

Indications, route, and dosage

Indications and dosage may vary. Check current literature for recommended protocol.
Trophoblastic tumors (choriocarcinoma, hydatidiform mole)
Adults: 15 to 30 mg P.O. or I.M. daily for 5 days. Repeat after 1 or more weeks, according to response or toxicity.
Tumors of head and neck, refractory lymphomas
Adults and children: High-dose methotrexate—up to 6 g/m² as an infusion over 6 to 12 hours.
Acute lymphoblastic and lymphatic leukemia
Adults and children: 3.3 mg/m² P.O., I.M., or I.V. daily for 4 to 6 weeks or until remission occurs; then 20 to 30 mg/m² P.O. or I.M. twice weekly or 2.5 mg/kg I.V. q 14 days.

Meningeal leukemia
Adults and children: 12 mg/m^2 intrathecally to a maximum dose of 15 mg q 2 to 5 days until CSF is normal. Use only vials of powder with no preservatives; dilute using 0.9% sodium chloride injection without preservatives or Elliot's B solution. Use only new vials of drug and diluent. Use immediately after reconstitution.

Burkitt's lymphoma (stage I or stage II)
Adults: 10 to 25 mg P.O. daily for 4 to 8 days with 1-week rest intervals.

Lymphosarcoma (stage III; non-Hodgkin's lymphoma)
Adults: 0.625 to 2.5 mg/kg daily P.O., I.M., or I.V.

Breast cancer
Women: 40 to 60 mg/m^2 I.V. as a single dose. Usually used in combination with other agents.

Mycosis fungoides (advanced)
Adults: 2.5 to 10 mg P.O. daily, 50 mg I.M. weekly, or 25 mg I.M. twice weekly.

Psoriasis (severe)
Adults: 10 to 25 mg P.O., I.M., or I.V. as single weekly dose.

Rheumatoid arthritis (severe, refractory)
Adults: 7.5 to 15 mg/week in divided doses.

Pharmacodynamics

Methotrexate exerts its cytotoxic activity by tightly binding with dihydrofolic acid reductase, an enzyme crucial to purine metabolism, resulting in inhibition of DNA, RNA, and protein synthesis.

Pharmacokinetics

Absorption: Methotrexate absorption across the GI tract appears to be dose related. Lower doses are essentially completely absorbed; absorption of larger doses is incomplete and variable. I.M. doses are absorbed completely. Peak serum levels are achieved 30 minutes to 2 hours after an I.M. dose and 1 to 4 hours after an oral dose.

Distribution: Methotrexate is distributed widely throughout the body, with the highest concentrations found in the kidneys, gallbladder, spleen, liver, and skin. The drug crosses the blood-brain barrier but does not achieve therapeutic levels in the CSF. Approximately 50% of the drug is bound to plasma proteins.

Metabolism: Methotrexate is metabolized only slightly in the liver.

Excretion: Methotrexate is excreted primarily into urine as unchanged drug. The elimination is biphasic, with an initial phase half-life of about 45 minutes and a terminal phase half-life of about 4 hours.

Contraindications and precautions

Methotrexate is a potentially toxic drug. The most common toxic effects involve rapidly dividing cells of the bone marrow and GI tract.

Methotrexate is contraindicated in pregnant patients because it may be fetotoxic. It is also contraindicated in nursing women because of the risk of serious adverse effects to the infant.

Use cautiously in patients with impaired renal, hepatic, or hematologic status because of the drug's adverse effects.

Administer by intrathecal injection with extreme caution. Large doses may cause seizures. Serum levels of the drug following intrathecal injection may be high enough to cause systemic toxicity.

Use with extreme caution in patients with peptic ulcer disease or ulcerative colitis.

Because the drug has the potential for both acute and chronic hepatotoxicity, use with extreme caution in patients with preexisting liver damage or impaired hepatic function. Chronic toxicity, characterized by hepatic fibrosis and cirrhosis, is potentially fatal. It is usually seen following long-term use (2 years or longer) and cumulative doses of 1.5 g.

Methotrexate therapy should be discontinued if the patient experiences pulmonary symptoms, such as a dry, nonproductive cough or evidence of a nonspecific pneumonitis. Fever, cough, dyspnea, hypoxemia, and radiologic evidence of a pulmonary infiltrate are typical findings.

Interactions

Concomitant use with probenecid increases the therapeutic and toxic effects of methotrexate by inhibiting renal tubular secretion of methotrexate; salicylates also increase the therapeutic and toxic effects of methotrexate by the same mechanism. Combined use with these drugs requires a lower dosage of methotrexate.

NSAIDs, sulfonamides, salicylates, and sulfonylureas may increase the therapeutic and toxic effects of methotrexate by displacing methotrexate from plasma proteins, increasing the concentrations of free methotrexate. Concurrent use of these agents with methotrexate should be avoided if possible.

Immunizations may not be effective when given during methotrexate therapy. Because of the risk of disseminated infections, live virus vaccines are generally not recommended during therapy.

Phenytoin serum levels may be decreased by chemotherapeutic regimens that employ methotrexate, resulting in an increased risk of seizures.

Effects on diagnostic tests

Methotrexate therapy may increase blood and urine concentrations of uric acid. Methotrexate may alter results of the laboratory assay for folate by inhibiting the organism used in the assay, thus interfering with the detection of folic acid deficiency.

Adverse reactions

CNS: *arachnoiditis within hours of intrathecal use;* subacute neurotoxicity may begin a few weeks later; necrotizing demyelinating leukoencephalopathy a few years later.
DERM: exposure to sun may aggravate psoriatic lesions, photosensitivity; urticaria, pruritus, hyperpigmentation, rash.
GI: stomatitis; diarrhea leading to *hemorrhagic enteritis* and *intestinal perforation;* nausea; vomiting; gingivitis; pharyngitis. *(Note:* Drug should be discontinued if diarrhea or ulcerative stomatitis occurs.)
GU: *tubular necrosis.*
HEMA: *bone marrow depression* (dose-limiting); *leukopenia* and *thrombocytopenia* (nadir occurring on day 7), anemia.
Hepatic: hepatic dysfunction leading to cirrhosis or hepatic fibrosis.
Metabolic: hyperuricemia.
Other: alopecia, *pulmonary interstitial infiltrates;* long-term use in children may cause osteoporosis.

---

*Canada only   †Off-label use   Italicized adverse reactions are life-threatening.

Overdose and treatment

Clinical manifestations of overdose include myelosuppression, anemia, nausea, vomiting, dermatitis, alopecia, and melena.

The antidote for the hematopoietic toxicity of methotrexate is leucovorin calcium, started within 1 hour after administration of methotrexate. The dosage of leucovorin should be high enough to produce plasma concentrations higher than those of methotrexate.

Special considerations

- Methotrexate may be given undiluted by I.V. push injection.
- Methotrexate can be diluted to a higher volume with 0.9% sodium chloride solution for I.V. infusion.
- Use reconstituted solutions of preservative-free drug within 24 hours after mixing.
- For intrathecal administration, use preservative-free formulations only. Dilute with unpreserved 0.9% sodium chloride solution and further dilute with either lactated Ringer's or Elliott's B solution, to a final concentration of 1 mg/ml.
- Dose modification may be required in presence of impaired hepatic or renal function, bone marrow depression, aplasia, leukopenia, thrombocytopenia, or anemia.
- Adverse GI effects include severe nausea and vomiting or stomatitis. Monitor patient for dehydration. These adverse reactions may require discontinuing the drug.
- Rash, redness, mouth ulcerations, or pulmonary adverse reactions may signal serious complications.
- Monitor uric acid levels.
- Monitor intake and output daily. Force fluids (2 to 3 liters daily).
- Alkalinize urine by giving sodium bicarbonate tablets to prevent precipitation of drug, especially with high doses. Maintain urine pH at more than 6.5. Reduce dose if BUN level is 20 to 30 mg/dl or serum creatinine level is 1.2 to 2 mg/dl. Discontinue drug if BUN level is more than 30 mg/dl or serum creatinine level is more than 2 mg/dl.

- Watch for increases in AST (formerly SGOT), ALT (formerly SGPT), and alkaline phosphatase levels, which may signal hepatic dysfunction.
- Methotrexate redistributes slowly from third-space compartments, such as ascitic fluid or pleural effusions. Slow redistribution can result in prolonged high blood levels of methotrexate and resultant toxicity. Before administering methotrexate to patients with significant third-space lesions, evacuate the fluid. Monitor plasma levels closely.
- Watch for bleeding (especially GI) and infection.
- Monitor temperature daily, and watch for cough, dyspnea, and cyanosis.
- Avoid all I.M. injections in patients with thrombocytopenia.
- Leucovorin rescue is necessary with high-dose (greater than 100 mg) protocols.

Information for the patient
- Emphasize importance of continuing medication despite nausea and vomiting. Advise patient to call immediately if vomiting occurs shortly after taking a dose.
- Encourage adequate fluid intake to increase urine output, to prevent nephrotoxicity, and to facilitate uric acid excretion.
- Warn patient to avoid alcoholic beverages during methotrexate therapy.
- Warn patient to avoid conception during and immediately after therapy because of possible abortion or congenital anomalies.
- Tell patient to avoid prolonged exposure to sunlight and to use a highly protective sunscreen when exposed to sunlight.
- Teach patient good mouth care to prevent superinfection of oral cavity.
- Advise patient that hair should grow back after treatment has ended.
- Recommend salicylate-free analgesics for pain relief or fever reduction.
- Tell patient to avoid exposure to persons with infections.
- Advise patient to report any unusual bruising or bleeding promptly.

---

thioguanine (6-thioguanine, 6-TG)
Lanvis, Thioguanine Tabloid
Pregnancy risk category: D

How supplied

Tablets (scored): 40 mg

Indications, route, and dosage

Indications and dosage may vary. Check current literature
for recommended protocol.

**Acute lymphoblastic and myelogenous leukemia, chronic granulocytic
leukemia**

Adults and children: Initially, 2 mg/kg/day P.O. (usually calculated to nearest 20 mg) or 75 to 100 mg/m^2/day P.O.; then, if
no toxic effects occur, increase gradually over 3 to 4 weeks to
3 mg/kg/day. Maintenance dosage is 2 to 3 mg/kg/day P.O.
or 100 mg/m^2/day P.O.

Pharmacodynamics

Thioguanine requires conversion intracellularly to its active
form to exert its cytotoxic activity. Acting as a false metabolite, thioguanine inhibits purine synthesis. Cross-resistance
exists between mercaptopurine and thioguanine.

Pharmacokinetics

Absorption: After an oral dose, the absorption of thioguanine
is incomplete and variable. The average bioavailability is
about 30%.

Distribution: Thioguanine distributes well into bone marrow
cells. The drug does not cross the blood-brain barrier to any
appreciable extent.

Metabolism: Thioguanine is extensively metabolized to a less
active form in the liver and other tissues.

Excretion: Plasma concentrations of thioguanine decrease in
a biphasic manner, with a half-life of about 15 minutes in
the initial phase and about 11 hours in the terminal phase.
Thioguanine is excreted in the urine, mainly as metabolites.

Contraindications and precautions

Thioguanine is contraindicated in patients with a history of resistance to previous therapy with the drug. Use with caution in patients with renal or hepatic dysfunction because of the potential for drug accumulation.

Interactions

None reported.

Effects on diagnostic tests

Hepatotoxic effects of thioguanine may cause elevations in ALT (formerly SGPT), AST (formerly SGOT), alkaline phosphatase, or bilirubin levels. Thioguanine therapy may increase blood and urine levels of uric acid.

Adverse reactions

GI: nausea, vomiting, stomatitis, diarrhea, anorexia.
HEMA: *bone marrow depression* (dose-limiting), *leukopenia,* anemia, *thrombocytopenia* (occurs slowly over 2 to 4 weeks).
Hepatic: hepatotoxicity, jaundice. *(Note:* Drug should be discontinued if jaundice occurs.)
Metabolic: hyperuricemia.

Overdose and treatment

Clinical signs of overdose include myelosuppression, nausea, vomiting, malaise, hypertension, and diaphoresis.

Treatment is usually supportive and includes transfusion of blood components and administration of antiemetics. Induction of emesis may be helpful if performed soon after ingestion.

Special considerations

- Total daily dose can be given at one time.
- Give dose between meals to facilitate complete absorption.
- Closely monitor liver function studies throughout therapy.
- Dose modification may be required in renal or hepatic dysfunction.
- Discontinue thioguanine if hepatotoxicity or hepatic tenderness occurs. Watch for jaundice; this may be reversed if thioguanine therapy is discontinued promptly.

- Monitor serum uric acid levels. Use oral hydration to prevent uric acid nephropathy. Alkalinize urine if serum uric acid levels are elevated.
- Monitor CBC daily during induction, then weekly during maintenance therapy.
- Drug is sometimes ordered as 6-thioguanine.
- Avoid all I.M. injections when platelet count is below 100,000/mm^3.

Information for the patient
- Emphasize importance of continuing medication despite nausea and vomiting.
- Tell patient to call promptly if vomiting occurs shortly after a dose is taken.
- Encourage adequate fluid intake to increase urine output and facilitate uric acid excretion.
- Advise patient to avoid exposure to persons with infections.
- Tell patient to discontinue the drug immediately if jaundice occurs.

trimetrexate glucuronate
Pregnancy risk category: C

How supplied
Injection: 25-mg vials

Indications, route, and dosage
Indications and dosage may vary. Check current literature for recommended protocol.
Adults: 30 mg/m^2 I.V. bolus daily for 21 days, administered with leucovorin (20 mg/m^2 I.V. or P.O. daily).

Pharmacodynamics
In vitro, the affinity of trimetrexate for *Pneumocystis* dihydrofolate reductase is about 1,500 times that of trimethoprim. Unlike methotrexate, trimetrexate is highly lipophilic and is passively taken up by and concentrated in protozoan cells.

Pharmacokinetics

Absorption: No data are currently available regarding oral bioavailability.

Distribution: Trimetrexate distributes rapidly after I.V. administration.

Metabolism: Trimetrexate is probably metabolized by the liver; at least two metabolites (one active) have been identified.

Excretion: Trimetrexate is excreted in bile and urine.

Contraindications and precautions

Because of the risk of potentially lethal trimetrexate-induced myelosuppression secondary to the drug's inhibition of dihydrofolate reductase, concomitant leucovorin therapy is essential in patients receiving trimetrexate. Other potentially myelosuppressive (including zidovudine) or nephrotoxic therapy should be discontinued during trimetrexate therapy but can be resumed as soon as treatment with trimetrexate and leucovorin is complete.

Interactions

None reported.

Effects on diagnostic tests

Information not available.

Adverse reactions

DERM: rash.

GI: mucositis, stomatitis, nausea, vomiting, diarrhea.

HEMA: *neutropenia, thrombocytopenia.*

Hepatic: *hepatotoxicity,* liver function test abnormalities.

Other: peripheral neuropathy, fever.

Overdose and treatment

Although no overdose information is available, clinical effects are expected to be similar to those of methotrexate. Methotrexate overdose produces myelosuppression, anemia, nausea, vomiting, dermatitis, alopecia, and melena.

Specific treatment information is unavailable, but levocovorin calcium would probably serve as an appropriate

---

treatment. Contact the manufacturer (Warner-Lambert Company) for further information.

Special considerations

- Trimetrexate glucuronate is an orphan drug available for hospital use to treat qualifying patients with *Pneumocystis carinii* pneumonia who have exhibited severe or life-threatening intolerance to both co-trimoxazole and pentamidine. Under the treatment protocol, patients are eligible to receive trimetrexate if they have an unequivocal diagnosis of *P. carinii* pneumonia; are human immunodeficiency virus (HIV)-positive by enzyme-linked immunosorbent assay (ELISA), HIV culture, or p24 core antigenemia (p24 gag proteinemia); have experienced a serious or life-threatening adverse reaction to conventional therapy (such as co-trimoxazole or pentamidine); and are age 12 or older. If laboratory confirmation of HIV infection has not been made before request for use of trimetrexate, a history of high-risk behavior for HIV infection (for example, homosexual or bisexual male, I.V. drug abuser, recipient of HIV-positive blood product, or sexual partner of an individual in one of these groups) will suffice.
- Avoid I.M. injections in patient with thrombocytopenia.
- Store intact vials in refrigerator.
- Trimetrexate is incompatible with chloride-containing solutions (including 0.9% sodium chloride solution). Only dextrose 5% in water is recommended for infusions.
- Dosage adjustments may be necessary in patients with altered hepatic or renal function.
- Leucovorin should be continued for 72 hours after the last dose of trimetrexate.

Information for the patient
Remind patient to avoid persons with infection during therapy.

Antineoplastics that alter hormone balance

---

aminoglutethimide

estramustine phosphate
sodium

flutamide

goserelin acetate

leuprolide acetate

megestrol acetate

mitotane

tamoxifen citrate

testolactone

trilostane

Antineoplastics that alter hormone balance attack cancer cells by disrupting the balance of naturally occurring factors that promote the tumor's growth. These drugs are especially useful in treating cancer because they inhibit neoplastic growth in specific tissues without causing widespread cytotoxicity.

Pharmacology

Drugs from several different pharmacologic classes are used to alter hormone balance. Aminoglutethimide, mitotane, and trilostane are adrenocortical suppressants with antisteroid actions. Estramustine, an estradiol-nitrogen mustard combination, exerts its hormonal effects on the prostate gland. The antiandrogen flutamide inhibits androgen uptake and binding. Goserelin and leuprolide are luteinizing hormone-releasing hormone (LHRH) analogs, which ultimately decrease testosterone levels. Synthetic sex hormones, such as megestrol and testolactone, counterbalance the tumor-stimulating effects of endogenous sex hormones. Tamoxifen is an estrogen antagonist.

Clinical indications and actions

The antineoplastics that alter hormone balance are used to treat breast, endometrial, prostate, and adrenocortical cancers; to stimulate ovulation; and to suppress adrenal function in patients with Cushing's syndrome or adrenal cancer. See the individual drugs discussed in this chapter for specific uses.

Overview of adverse reactions

Many adverse reactions to antineoplastic agents that alter hormone balance are extensions of the hormonal activity of these agents. For example, they may cause gynecomastia, breast tenderness, hot flashes, sexual dysfunction (such as decreased libido and impotence), or vaginal discharge or bleeding. Other common adverse reactions include GI distress, such as nausea, vomiting, anorexia, and diarrhea, and CNS, cardiovascular, hematologic, dermatologic, and fluid and electrolyte disturbances. Specific adverse reactions vary with the antineoplastic prescribed.

Special considerations

- Administer the drug exactly as prescribed and according to protocol. Improper administration of some drugs can cause an embolus.
- Monitor hydration and nutritional status if nausea or vomiting occurs. Administer an antiemetic before meals, if prescribed.
- Regularly assess for signs of fluid retention, such as sudden weight gain, edema, and crackles in the lungs. Expect to reduce fluid intake, as prescribed.
- Monitor for signs of thromboembolic and other cardiovascular complications.
- Take safety precautions if adverse CNS reactions occur. For example, place the bed in a low position, keep the bed rails up, and supervise ambulation.
- Monitor the results of liver function studies; serum calcium, sodium, and potassium levels; blood glucose and triglyceride levels; WBC and platelet counts; prothrom-

bin time; and other laboratory tests, as ordered for the specific agent.

Information for the patient
- Advise patient of the prescribed drug's potential effects on sexual characteristics and functioning. Discuss patient concerns and provide emotional support.
- Teach patient to recognize and report signs of fluid retention and other adverse reactions.
- If appropriate, inform patient that tumor flare may occur, but can be managed with analgesics until it subsides.
- Urge patient to return promptly for follow-up blood tests and other studies, as prescribed.

aminoglutethimide
Cytadren
Pregnancy risk category: D

How supplied
Tablets: 250 mg

Indications, route, and dosage
Indications and dosage may vary. Check current literature for recommended protocol.
Adrenal hyperplasia from ectopic corticotropin–producing tumors, †medical adrenalectomy in postmenopausal metastatic breast cancer, †prostate cancer, suppression of adrenal function in Cushing's syndrome
Adults: Initiate therapy at 250 mg P.O. b.i.d. or t.i.d. for 2 weeks. Maintenance dose is 250 mg P.O. q.i.d. at 6-hour intervals. Dosage may be increased in increments of 250 mg daily q 1 to 2 weeks to a maximum total daily dose of 2 g.

Pharmacodynamics
Aminoglutethimide interferes with the enzymatic conversion of cholesterol to delta-5-pregnenolone, effectively inhibiting the synthesis of corticosteroids, androgens, and

---

estrogens. By suppressing the adrenal glands, aminoglutethimide inhibits the growth of tumors that need estrogen to thrive.

Pharmacokinetics

Absorption: Aminoglutethimide is well absorbed across the GI tract after oral administration.
Distribution: Aminoglutethimide is distributed widely into body tissues.
Metabolism: Aminoglutethimide is metabolized extensively in the liver.
Excretion: Aminoglutethimide and its metabolites are primarily eliminated through the kidneys, mostly as unchanged drug.

Contraindications and precautions

Aminoglutethimide is contraindicated in patients with a history of hypersensitivity to the drug or to glutethimide because cross-sensitivity may exist.

Aminoglutethimide should be used cautiously in elderly patients because they may be more sensitive to its adverse CNS reactions, and in patients with serious infections or hypothyroidism because the drug may worsen the symptoms of these disorders.

Interactions

Concomitant use of aminoglutethimide with dexamethasone decreases the half-life and therapeutic effect of dexamethasone by increasing the metabolism of dexamethasone.

By a similar mechanism, aminoglutethimide may diminish the effects of warfarin, theophylline, digitoxin, and medroxyprogesterone.

Effects on diagnostic tests

Aminoglutethimide therapy may decrease plasma cortisol, serum thyroxine, and urinary aldosterone levels, and may increase serum alkaline phosphatase, AST (formerly SGOT), and thyroid-stimulating hormone concentrations.

Adverse reactions

CNS: drowsiness, headache, dizziness, nystagmus.
CV: hypotension, tachycardia.
DERM: morbilliform skin rash, pruritus, urticaria.
Endocrine: adrenal insufficiency, masculinization, hirsutism, hypothyroidism.
GI: nausea, vomiting, anorexia, cholestatic jaundice.
HEMA: transient leukopenia, *severe pancytopenia*.
Other: fever, myalgia, hypothyroidism.

Overdose and treatment

Clinical manifestations of overdose include exaggerated skin rash, hypotension, nausea, and vomiting.

Treatment usually is supportive and includes induction of emesis, gastric lavage, administration of antiemetics, and symptomatic treatment of abnormal vital signs. Aminoglutethimide is removable by dialysis.

Special considerations

- Give in divided doses, two to three times a day, to reduce the incidence of nausea and vomiting.
- Most adverse effects will decrease in incidence and severity after the first 2 to 6 weeks of therapy because metabolism of drug accelerates with continued use.
- Some clinicians advocate routine hydrocortisone supplementation as glucocorticoid replacement in patients with metastatic breast cancer.
- Adrenal hypofunction may develop under stressful conditions such as surgery, trauma, or acute illness. Additional steroids may be required to ensure a normal response to stress.
- Aminoglutethimide therapy does not require gradually tapered withdrawal because the adrenal cortex rapidly returns to normal responsiveness following cessation of therapy.
- Up to 50% of patients will require mineralocorticoid replacement with fludrocortisone at a dosage of 0.1 mg daily or three times per week.
- Monitor blood pressure frequently.

• Perform baseline hematologic studies and monitor CBC periodically. Also monitor thyroid function studies because aminoglutethimide may decrease thyroid hormone production.

Information for the patient
• Emphasize the importance of continuing drug therapy despite nausea and vomiting, which usually subside with time.
• Warn patient that drowsiness may occur. Tell him to avoid hazardous activities that require alertness until sedative effect subsides. Patients usually develop tolerance within a month.
• If a skin rash develops when starting therapy, tell patient to call if it persists for 5 to 8 days. Therapy may be discontinued temporarily until rash clears.
• Advise patient to stand up slowly to avoid dizziness.

Geriatric use
Elderly patients are more sensitive to adverse CNS reactions and are more likely to be lethargic. Safety precautions are recommended.

estramustine phosphate sodium
Emcyt
Pregnancy risk category: C

How supplied

Capsules: 140 mg

Indications, route, and dosage

Indications and dosage may vary. Check literature for recommended protocol.
Palliative treatment of metastatic or progressive cancer of the prostate gland
Men: 10 to 16 mg/kg P.O. in three to four divided doses. Usual dosage is 14 mg/kg daily. Therapy should continue for up to 3 months and, if successful, be maintained as long as the patient responds.

Pharmacodynamics

The exact mechanism of action is unclear. However, the estrogenic portion of the molecule may act as a carrier of the drug to facilitate selective uptake by tumor cells with estradiol hormone receptors, such as those in the prostate gland. At that point, the nitrogen mustard portion of the drug acts as an alkylating agent.

Pharmacokinetics

Absorption: After oral administration, about 75% of a dose is absorbed across the GI tract.
Distribution: Estramustine distributes widely into body tissues.
Metabolism: Estramustine is extensively metabolized in the liver.
Excretion: Estramustine and its metabolites are eliminated primarily in feces, with a small amount excreted in urine. The terminal plasma elimination half-life is about 20 hours.

Contraindications and precautions

Estramustine is contraindicated in patients with a history of hypersensitivity to the drug or to estradiol or mechlorethamine; cross-sensitivity may occur. The drug is also contraindicated in patients with peptic ulcers, severe liver disease, cardiac disease, or impaired bone marrow function because it may worsen these conditions.

Because of the drug's cardiovascular toxicity, it should be used cautiously in patients with thromboembolic disorders, cerebrovascular disorders, or coronary artery disease.

Interactions

Concomitant use of estramustine with anticoagulants may decrease the anticoagulant effect by an unknown mechanism; increase dosage of anticoagulants given concurrently.

Effects on diagnostic tests

Estramustine therapy may increase norepinephrine-induced platelet aggregability. A reduced response to the metyrapone test may occur during therapy with estramustine. Glucose tolerance may be decreased.

Adverse reactions

CNS: anxiety, headache, emotional lability.
CV: *MI, CVA,* edema, *pulmonary emboli,* thrombophlebitis, *CHF,* hypertension.
DERM: rash, pruritus.
GI: nausea and vomiting (dose-limiting), diarrhea, anorexia. *(Note:* Drug should be discontinued if intractable GI toxicity occurs.)
HEMA: *leukopenia, thrombocytopenia,* hypercalcemia.
Other: painful gynecomastia and breast tenderness, thinning of hair, hyperglycemia, infertility, azoospermia.

Overdose and treatment

Clinical manifestations of overdose include headache, nausea, vomiting, and myelosuppression.

Treatment is usually supportive and includes induction of emesis, gastric lavage, transfusion of blood components, and appropriate symptomatic therapy. Hematologic monitoring should continue for at least 6 weeks.

Special considerations

Besides those relevant to all alkylating agents, consider the following recommendations.
- Estramustine may be administered with meals or antacids to reduce the incidence of GI upset. However, calcium-rich foods may impair absorption.
- Store capsules in refrigerator.
- Phenothiazines can be used to treat nausea and vomiting.
- Monitor blood pressure at baseline and routinely during therapy. Estramustine may cause hypertension.
- Estramustine may exaggerate preexisting peripheral edema or CHF. Weight gain should be monitored regularly in these patients.
- Monitor glucose tolerance periodically throughout estramustine therapy.
- Patient may continue estramustine as long as he's responding favorably. Some patients have taken the drug for more than 3 years.

Information for the patient

- Emphasize importance of continuing medication despite nausea and vomiting.
- Advise patient to call immediately if vomiting occurs shortly after a dose is taken.
- Because of the possibility of mutagenic effects, advise couples of childbearing age to use contraceptive measures.

Geriatric use

Use with caution in elderly patients, who are more likely to have vascular disorders, because the use of estrogen is associated with vascular complications.

flutamide
Eulexin

Pregnancy risk category: D

How supplied

Capsules: 125 mg

Indication, route, and dosage

Treatment of metastatic prostatic cancer (stage D2) in combination with LHRH analogs, such as leuprolide acetate
Men: 250 mg P.O. q 8 hours.

Pharmacodynamics

Flutamide inhibits androgen uptake or prevents binding of androgens in nucleus of cells within target tissues. Prostatic cancer is known to be androgen-sensitive.

Pharmacokinetics

Absorption: Rapid and complete absorption occurs after oral administration.
Distribution: Studies in animals show that flutamide concentrates in the prostate gland. Flutamide and its major active metabolite are about 95% protein bound.
Metabolism: The metabolism of flutamide is rapid, with at least six metabolites identified. Over 97% of the drug is metabolized within 1 hour of administration.

Excretion: Over 95% of a dose is excreted in the urine.

Contraindications and precautions

Flutamide is contraindicated in patients allergic to the drug.

Animal studies indicate that flutamide may harm the fetus if administered to a pregnant patient.

Interactions

None reported.

Effects on diagnostic tests

Elevation of plasma testosterone and estradiol levels has been reported. Serum ALT (formerly SGPT), AST (formerly SGOT), bilirubin, and creatinine levels may be increased.

Adverse reactions

CNS: loss of libido, drowsiness, confusion, nervousness.
CV: edema, hypertension.
DERM: rash, photosensitivity.
GI: diarrhea, nausea, vomiting.
GU: impotence.
Metabolic: gynecomastia, elevation of hepatic enzymes, hepatitis.
Other: hot flashes.

Overdose and treatment

No experience with overdose in humans has been reported. Dosages as high as 1,500 mg daily have been given for 36 weeks without serious adverse effects.

Special considerations

- Flutamide must be taken continuously with the agent used for medical castration (such as leuprolide acetate) to produce full benefit of therapy. Leuprolide suppresses testosterone production, and flutamide inhibits testosterone action at the cellular level. Together they can impair the growth of androgen-responsive tumors.
- Perform periodic liver tests in patients receiving prolonged therapy with flutamide.

Information for the patient

- Tell patient not to discontinue either leuprolide or fluta-mide without medical approval.
- Explain to patient that some symptoms may worsen initially before they improve.

goserelin acetate
Zoladex

Pregnancy risk category: X

How supplied

Implant: 3.6 mg

Indications, route, and dosage

Palliative treatment of advanced prostate cancer
Men: One implant S.C. into the upper abdominal wall q 28 days.

Pharmacodynamics

Chronic administration of goserelin, an LHRH, acts on the pituitary to decrease the release of follicle-stimulating hor-mone and luteinizing hormone. In males, the result is dra-matically lowered serum testosterone levels.

Pharmacokinetics

Absorption: Goserelin is slowly absorbed from the implanta-tion site. Drug levels peak in 12 to 15 days.
Distribution: No information available.
Metabolism: No information available.
Excretion: Elimination half-life is about 4.2 hours in patients with normal renal function. Substantial renal impairment prolongs half-life, but this does not appear to increase the in-cidence of adverse effects.

Contraindications and precautions

The manufacturer states that goserelin is contraindicated during pregnancy.

---

*Canada only †Off-label use Italicized adverse reactions are life-threatening.

Initially, LHRH analogs such as goserelin may cause a worsening of the symptoms of prostate cancer because the drug initially increases serum testosterone levels. A few patients may experience increased bone pain. Rarely, disease exacerbation (spinal cord compression or ureteral obstruction) has occurred.

Interactions

None reported.

Effects on diagnostic tests

Serum testosterone levels increase during the first week of therapy and then decrease. Serum acid phosphatase levels may increase initially and will decrease by week 4.

Adverse reactions

CNS: lethargy, pain (worsened in the first 30 days), dizziness, insomnia, anxiety, depression, headache, chills, fever.
CV: edema, *CHF, arrhythmias, CVA,* hypertension, *MI,* peripheral vascular disorder, chest pain.
DERM: rash, sweating.
EENT: upper respiratory infection.
GI: nausea, vomiting, diarrhea, constipation, ulcer.
GU: decreased erections, dysuria, renal insufficiency, urinary obstruction, urinary tract infection.
HEMA: anemia.
Other: hot flashes, sexual dysfunction, gout, hyperglycemia, weight increase, breast swelling and tenderness.

Overdose and treatment

No information is available regarding accidental or intentional overdosage of goserelin in humans. In animal studies, doses up to 1 mg/kg/day did not produce nonendocrine-related symptoms.

Special considerations

• The implant comes in a preloaded syringe. If the package is damaged, do not use the syringe. Make sure that the drug is visible in the translucent chamber of the syringe.

- Goserelin should be given every 28 days, always under direct supervision of a doctor. Local anesthesia may be given before the injection.
- Administer the drug in the upper abdominal wall using aseptic technique. After cleaning the area with an alcohol wipe (and injecting a local anesthetic), stretch the patient's skin with one hand while grasping the barrel of the syringe with the other. Insert the needle into the subcutaneous fat; then change the needle direction to parallel the abdominal wall. Push the needle in until the hub touches the patient's skin; then withdraw it about ¹/₂" (1 cm), which creates room for the drug to be injected, before depressing the plunger completely.
- After inserting the needle, do not aspirate because blood will be seen instantly in the chamber if a large vessel is penetrated (a new syringe and injection site will be needed).
- Store the drug at room temperature, not to exceed 77° F (25° C).

Information for the patient
Advise the patient to report every 28 days for a new implant. However, a delay of a couple of days is permissible.

leuprolide acetate
Lupron, Lupron Depot

Pregnancy risk category: X

How supplied
Injection: 5 mg/ml in 2.8-ml multiple-dose vials
Suspension for depot injection: 3.75 mg, 7.5 mg

Indications, route, and dosage
Indications and dosage may vary. Check current literature for recommended protocol.
Management of advanced prostate cancer
Men: 7.5 mg I.M. (depot injection) once monthly or 1 mg S.C. daily.

Treatment of endometriosis

Women: 3.75 mg I.M. (depot injection) once monthly for a maximum of 6 months.

Pharmacodynamics

Leuprolide is a synthetic LHRH analog. It inhibits gonadotropin secretion and androgen or estrogen synthesis. Because of this effect, leuprolide may inhibit the growth of hormone-dependent tumors.

Because leuprolide lowers levels of sex hormones, it causes a decrease in the size of endometrial implants, resulting in decreased dysmenorrhea and pelvic pain in women with endometriosis.

Pharmacokinetics

Absorption: Leuprolide is a polypeptide molecule that is destroyed in the GI tract. After S.C. administration, the drug is rapidly, and essentially completely, absorbed.

Distribution: Distribution in humans has not been determined; however, it is suggested that high concentrations distribute into kidney, liver, pineal, and pituitary tissue. Approximately 7% to 15% of a dose is bound to plasma proteins.

Metabolism: The metabolic fate of leuprolide is unclear, but it may be metabolized in the anterior pituitary and hypothalamus, similar to endogenous gonadotropin-releasing hormone.

Excretion: The plasma elimination half-life has been reported to be about 3 hours.

Contraindications and precautions

Leuprolide is contraindicated in patients with hypersensitivity to gonadotropin hormone-releasing hormone (GNRH) and GNRH analogs, in women with undiagnosed vaginal bleeding, and in pregnant patients.

Use with caution in patients who are sensitive to benzyl alcohol, a preservative used in some formulations.

Interactions

None reported.

---

*Canada only   †Off-label use   Italicized adverse reactions are life-threatening.

Effects on diagnostic tests

Serum acid phosphatase and testosterone levels initially increase, then decrease with continued therapy.

Adverse reactions

CNS: dizziness, numbness, headache, blurred vision, muscle pain.
CV: angina, *MI, arrhythmias, CHF.*
DERM: pruritus, rash.
Endocrine: hot flashes, breast tenderness, gynecomastia.
GI: nausea, vomiting, constipation, anorexia.
GU: infertility, impaired spermatogenesis.
Local: redness and induration at injection site.
Other: alopecia, *pulmonary embolus,* peripheral edema, decreased libido, transient bone pain during first week of treatment.

Overdose and treatment

No information available.

Special considerations

- Use a 22G needle for injection.
- When treating endometriosis, administer for a maximum of 6 months. Safety and efficacy of retreatment is unknown.
- Discard solution if particulate matter is visible or if the solution is discolored.
- Erythema or induration may develop at injection site.
- When used to treat prostate cancer, leuprolide may produce worsening of signs and symptoms of disease during the first 1 to 2 weeks of therapy. Temporary paresthesia and weakness may occur during the first week of therapy.
- Measure serum testosterone and acid phosphatase levels before and during therapy.
- No unusual adverse effects have been observed in patients who received 20 mg daily for 2 years.

Information for the patient

- Reassure patient that bone pain is transient and will disappear after about 1 week.

- Tell patient that he may experience temporary burning, itching, and swelling at the injection site. Tell patient to report persistent reactions.
- Advise patient to continue taking medication even if he experiences a sense of well-being.

megestrol acetate
Megace, Pallace

Pregnancy risk category: X

How supplied

Tablets: 20 mg, 40 mg

Indications, route, and dosage

Indications and dosage may vary. Check current literature for recommended protocol.
Breast cancer
Women: 40 mg P.O. q.i.d.
Endometrial cancer
Women: 10 to 80 mg P.O. q.i.d.
Cachexia caused by acquired immunodeficiency syndrome (AIDS) or neoplastic disease
Adults: 80 mg P.O. q.i.d.

Pharmacodynamics

Megestrol inhibits growth and causes regression of progestin-sensitive breast and endometrial cancer tissue by an unknown mechanism.

Pharmacokinetics

Absorption: Megestrol is well absorbed across the GI tract after oral administration.
Distribution: Megestrol appears to be stored in fatty tissue and is highly bound to plasma proteins.
Metabolism: Megestrol is completely metabolized in the liver.
Excretion: The metabolites are eliminated primarily through the kidneys.

Contraindications and precautions

Megestrol is contraindicated in patients with known hypersensitivity to progestins; in patients with a history of thromboembolic disorder because the drug may be associated with thromboembolic disease; in patients with severe hepatic disease because drug accumulation may occur; in patients with undiagnosed abnormal vaginal bleeding because drug may stimulate growth of some tumors; and in pregnant or breastfeeding patients because of the potential for adverse effects on the fetus or neonate.

Megestrol should be used cautiously in patients with conditions that might be aggravated by fluid and electrolyte retention, such as cardiac or renal disease, epilepsy, or migraine. Caution is also advised in administering the drug to diabetic patients because decreased glucose tolerance may occur. Use cautiously in patients with a history of mental depression because megestrol may worsen depression.

Interactions

Concomitant use with bromocriptine may cause amenorrhea or galactorrhea, thus interfering with the action of bromocriptine. Concurrent use of these drugs is not recommended.

Effects on diagnostic tests

Pregnanediol excretion may decrease; serum alkaline phosphatase and amino acid concentrations may increase. Glucose tolerance has been shown to decrease in a small percentage of patients receiving megestrol.

Adverse reactions

CV: thrombophlebitis.
GI: nausea, vomiting.
Other: carpal tunnel syndrome, alopecia.

Overdose and treatment

No information available.

Special considerations

- Glucose tolerance may be altered in diabetic patients. Monitor blood glucose carefully and adjust antidiabetic medication accordingly.
- Some patients using progestins may experience gingival hyperplasia or bleeding gums. Good oral hygiene and regular visits to the dentist may prevent further complications.
- Cachexia has been treated with high doses (800 to 1,600 mg daily) of the drug in some studies. The use of high-dose therapy is associated with an increase in incidence and severity of adverse reactions, such as CHF, elevated blood pressure, dyspnea, hyperpnea, and GI intolerance.

Information for the patient

Advise female patients to use an effective nonhormonal form of contraception. Explain the risks of progestin therapy on a developing fetus, and advise her to call the doctor if she suspects that she is pregnant.

mitotane
Lysodren

Pregnancy risk category: C

How supplied

Tablets (scored): 500 mg

Indications, route, and dosage

Indications and dosage may vary. Check current literature for recommended protocol.

Inoperable adrenocortical cancer

Adults: Initially, 1 to 6 g P.O. daily in divided doses t.i.d. or q.i.d. Increase to 9 to 10 g daily as tolerated. If severe adverse reactions appear, reduce dosage until maximum tolerated dosage is achieved (varies from 2 to 16 g daily but is usually 8 to 10 g daily).

Cushing's syndrome

Adults: 1 to 12 g P.O. daily in divided doses; maintenance dosage ranges from 500 mg twice weekly to 2 g daily.

---

*Canada only   †Off-label use   Italicized adverse reactions are life-threatening.

Pharmacodynamics

The exact mechanism of mitotane's activity is unclear. Possibly, a metabolite binds to mitochondrial proteins in the adrenal cortex, resulting in cell death.

Mitotane also inhibits the production of corticosteroids and alters extra-adrenal metabolism of endogenous and exogenous steroids.

Pharmacokinetics

Absorption: After oral administration, 35% to 40% of a dose is absorbed across the GI tract.
Distribution: Mitotane is widely distributed in body tissue; fatty tissue is the primary storage site. Slow release of mitotane from fatty tissue into the plasma occurs after the drug is discontinued. A metabolite of mitotane has been detected in CSF.
Metabolism: Mitotane is metabolized in the liver and other tissue.
Excretion: Mitotane and its metabolites are excreted in urine and bile. The plasma elimination half-life is reported to be 18 to 159 days.

Contraindications and precautions

Mitotane is contraindicated in patients with a history of hypersensitivity to the drug. It should be used cautiously in patients with impaired liver function; the drug may accumulate in the body because of impaired metabolism.

Interactions

When used concomitantly, mitotane may decrease the effect of barbiturates, coumarin anticoagulants, and phenytoin through the induction of hepatic microsomal enzymes, increasing the metabolism of these agents to inactive compounds. Concomitant use with CNS depressants can cause additive CNS depression. Spironolactone may block the actions of mitotane.

Effects on diagnostic tests

Mitotane therapy may decrease concentrations of urinary 17-hydroxycorticosteroids, plasma cortisol, protein-bound iodine, and serum uric acid.

Adverse reactions

CNS: depression; somnolence; vertigo; brain damage and dysfunction in long-term, high-dose therapy; fatigue.
CV: flushing.
DERM: maculopapular rash, pruritus, pigmentation, dermatitis.
GI: severe nausea, vomiting, diarrhea, anorexia.
GU: *hemorrhagic cystitis,* hematuria.
Metabolic: adrenal insufficiency.
Other: blurred vision, diplopia, fever.

  Note: Drug should be discontinued if patient suffers from shock, severe trauma, infection, or another condition that would be adversely affected by adrenocortical insufficiency.

Overdose and treatment

Clinical manifestations of overdose include vomiting, weakness, numbness of extremities, diarrhea, apprehension, and excitement.

  Treatment is usually supportive and includes administration of activated charcoal and a saline cathartic, induction of emesis with ipecac, intestinal lavage with mannitol 20%, and appropriate symptomatic therapy.

Special considerations

- Mitotane can be administered with or without food in the stomach. Avoid administering the drug with a fatty meal because the drug distributes mostly to body fat.
- To reduce nausea, give an antiemetic before administering mitotane.
- Dosage may be reduced if GI or skin reactions are severe.
- Dose modification may be required in patients with hepatic disease.
- Obese patients may need higher dosage and may have longer-lasting adverse reactions, because drug distributes mostly to body fat.

---

*Canada only   †Off-label use   Italicized adverse reactions are life-threatening.

- Evaluate efficacy by reduction in pain, weakness, anorexia, and tumor mass.
- Monitor for symptoms of hepatotoxicity.
- Mitotane should not be used in a patient with shock or trauma. Use of corticosteroids may avoid acute adrenocortical insufficiency.
- Glucocorticoid therapy is usually required. During periods of physiologic stress (such as infection or surgery), glucocorticoid dosage should be increased.
- Monitor behavioral and neurologic signs daily throughout therapy.
- Adequate trial is at least 3 months, but therapy can continue if clinical benefits are observed.

Information for the patient
- Tell patient it is important to continue medication despite nausea and vomiting.
- Warn patient to avoid alcoholic beverages after taking a dose of medication because excessive drowsiness may occur.
- Tell patient drug may cause drowsiness. Patient should use caution when performing activities that require mental alertness.
- Tell patient to call immediately if vomiting occurs shortly after taking a dose.

tamoxifen citrate
Nolvadex, Nolvadex-D*, Tamofen*
Pregnancy risk category: D

How supplied
Tablets: 10 mg, 20 mg
Tablets (enteric coated): 20 mg*

Indications, route, and dosage
Indications and dosage may vary. Check current literature for recommended protocol.
Advanced postmenopausal breast cancer
Women: 10 to 20 mg P.O. b.i.d.

Pharmacodynamics

The exact mechanism of action is unclear. Tamoxifen may exert its cytotoxic action by blocking estrogen receptors within tumor cells that require estrogen to thrive. The estrogen receptor–tamoxifen complex may be translocated into the nucleus of the tumor cell, where it inhibits DNA synthesis.

Pharmacokinetics

Absorption: Tamoxifen appears to be well absorbed across the GI tract after oral administration.
Distribution: Tamoxifen is distributed widely into total body water.
Metabolism: Tamoxifen is metabolized extensively in the liver to several metabolites.
Excretion: Tamoxifen and its metabolites are excreted primarily in feces, mostly as metabolites. The drug has a distribution phase half-life of 7 to 14 hours. Secondary peak plasma levels occur 4 days after a dose, probably because of enterohepatic circulation. The terminal elimination half-life is more than 7 days.

Contraindications and precautions

Tamoxifen is contraindicated in the first 4 months of pregnancy because of the potential for fetal harm. Use cautiously in patients with preexisting leukopenia and thrombocytopenia.

Interactions

Tamoxifen may potentiate the hypoprothrombinemic effect of warfarin. When initiating tamoxifen therapy in patients receiving warfarin, monitor patient and prothrombin time closely. Adjust anticoagulant dosage accordingly.

Effects on diagnostic tests

Tamoxifen therapy may increase concentrations of serum calcium. This effect usually occurs in patients with bone metastases.

Adverse reactions

CNS: headache, dizziness, depression, confusion.
CV: *thrombosis.*
DERM: rash, photosensitivity.
EENT: blurred vision, decreased visual acuity, corneal changes.
GI: nausea, vomiting, anorexia.
GU: vaginal discharge and bleeding.
HEMA: transient fall in WBC or platelet counts.
Metabolic: *hypercalcemia.*
Other: temporary bone or tumor pain, hot flashes, brief exacerbation of pain from osseous metastases.

Overdose and treatment

No information available.

Special considerations

- Initial adverse reactions (increased bone pain) may mimic a "disease flare."
- Analgesics are indicated to relieve pain.
- Adverse reactions are usually minor and are well tolerated. They can usually be controlled by dosage reduction.
- Monitor WBC and platelet counts.
- Monitor serum calcium levels. Drug may compound hypercalcemia related to bone metastases.
- Tamoxifen acts as an antiestrogen. Best results occur in patients with estrogen-receptor-positive tumors.
- Tamoxifen is also used to treat breast cancer in men, advanced ovarian cancer in women, and metastatic melanoma (in combination therapy).

Information for the patient
- Emphasize importance of continuing medication despite nausea and vomiting.
- Tell patient to call promptly if vomiting occurs shortly after a dose is taken.
- Reassure patient that acute exacerbation of bone pain during tamoxifen therapy usually indicates drug will produce good response.

---

testolactone
Teslac

Pregnancy risk category: C

How supplied

Tablets: 50 mg

Indications, route, and dosage

Dosage and indications may vary. Check current literature
for recommended protocol.
Advanced postmenopausal breast cancer
Women: 250 mg P.O. q.i.d.

Pharmacodynamics

The exact mechanism of action is unclear. Testolactone's
cytotoxic activity may result from depressed ovarian function that follows inhibition of pituitary gonadotropin synthesis or prevention of steroid action on tumor cells, which
the cell requires for survival.

Pharmacokinetics

Absorption: Testolactone is well absorbed across the GI tract
after oral administration.
Distribution: Testolactone is widely distributed into total body
water.
Metabolism: Testolactone is extensively metabolized in the
liver.
Excretion: Testolactone and its metabolites are excreted primarily in urine.

Contraindications and precautions

Testolactone is contraindicated in the treatment of breast
cancer in males and in premenopausal women because of
the potential for adverse hormonal effects.
    Use cautiously in patients with hypercalcemia and cardio-
vascular disease.

---

*Canada only   †Off-label use   Italicized adverse reactions are life-threatening.

Interactions

None reported.

Effects on diagnostic tests

Testolactone therapy may increase concentrations of serum calcium, urinary creatinine, and urinary 17-ketosteroids.

Adverse reactions

CNS: paresthesias.
CV: hypertension, orthostatic hypotension.
DERM: maculopapular rash, erythema.
GI: nausea, vomiting, anorexia, glossitis, diarrhea.
Metabolic: *hypercalcemia.*
Other: edema, hot flashes.

Overdose and treatment

No information available.

Special considerations

- Adequate trial is 3 months. Reassure patient that therapeutic response isn't immediate.
- Monitor fluids and electrolytes, especially calcium levels.
- Immobilized patients are prone to hypercalcemia. Exercise may prevent it. Force fluids to aid calcium excretion.
- Treat hypercalcemia with generous hydration; obtain calcium levels before and during therapy.
- Higher-than-recommended doses do not increase incidence of remission.
- Drug does not cause virilization when used at recommended doses.

Information for the patient

- Emphasize importance of continuing testolactone therapy despite nausea and vomiting.
- Tell patient to call promptly if vomiting occurs shortly after a dose is taken.

---

trilostane
Modrastane

Pregnancy Risk Category: X

How supplied

Capsules: 30 mg, 60 mg

Indications, route, and dosage

Indications and dosage may vary. Check literature for recommended protocol.

Adrenocortical hyperfunction in Cushing's syndrome
Adults: 30 mg P.O. q.i.d. initially. May be increased q 3 to 4 days to maximum of 480 mg daily.

Pharmacodynamics

Trilostane reversibly lowers elevated circulating levels of glucocorticoids by inhibiting the enzyme that converts biologically inactive steroids to biologically active forms.

Pharmacokinetics

Absorption: Although trilostane is absorbed readily from the GI tract, the rate and extent of absorption vary greatly among individuals.
Distribution: Trilostane may be distributed widely into most tissues, with highest concentrations in the adrenal glands, liver, lungs, and kidneys.
Metabolism: Hepatic metabolism of trilostane produces at least five metabolites. The major one, 17-ketotrilostane, is about twice as effective as the parent drug at enzyme inhibition.
Excretion: Unknown.

Contraindications and precautions

Trilostane is contraindicated in patients with severe renal or hepatic disease. It also should not be used in women of childbearing age unless pregnancy has been ruled out and an effective nonhormonal contraceptive is used.

Trilostane should be used cautiously in patients receiving other drugs that suppress adrenal function. For patients

---

with Cushing's syndrome, the manufacturer recommends hospitalization from the initiation of trilostane therapy to the achievement of a stable dosage regimen.

Interactions

Concomitant use of a drug that suppresses adrenal function, such as aminoglutethimide or mitotane, with trilostane may cause severe adrenocortical hypofunction.

Because of its effects on aldosterone formation, trilostane may decrease urinary potassium excretion. Trilostane will reduce the potassium loss caused by drugs, such as thiazide or loop diuretics. It also may normalize potassium levels in hypokalemic patients, requiring discontinuation of potassium supplements.

Effects on diagnostic tests

Trilostane, a synthetic steroid, may interfere with several tests that measure steroid levels. In tests that use fluorometric methods, trilostane may produce falsely high levels of urine or serum 11-hydroxycorticosteroids, particularly in urine samples. In tests that use radioimmunoassay methods (recommended during trilostane therapy), the drug may interfere with accurate determination of estrogen concentrations. A highly sensitive and specific antiserum may minimize this effect.

Adverse reactions

CNS: headache.
CV: orthostatic hypotension.
DERM: flushing, rash.
EENT: burning of oral and nasal membranes.
GI: diarrhea, upset stomach, nausea, flatulence, bloating.
Metabolic: hyperkalemia.
Other: fever, fatigue, hot flashes.

Overdose and treatment

Clinical manifestations of overdose include lethargy, confusion, hypotension, and possibly hyperkalemia.

After recent ingestion, emesis or gastric lavage is used to empty the stomach. Subsequent treatment includes close monitoring of plasma adrenal steroid levels for several days, treatment of adrenal insufficiency, and replacement dosages of a corticosteroid.

Special considerations

- Expect to see a therapeutic response at dosages below 360 mg/day. Although rare, dosages up to 960 mg/day have been used.
- Monitor blood pressure periodically, particularly noting orthostatic hypotension. Concomitant antihypertensive therapy may be adjusted or temporarily discontinued. A mineralocorticoid, such as fludrocortisone, may be prescribed to treat orthostatic hypotension.
- Monitor serum potassium levels periodically, observing for an increase. Consider temporarily withholding potassium supplements during trilostane therapy.
- Trilostane may prevent normal response to physiologic stress. Therefore, it may need to be discontinued temporarily if patient develops a severe illness or must undergo surgery.

Information for the patient

- Explain that the drug does not cure the underlying disease.
- Review the signs and symptoms of adrenal insufficiency. Advise patient to call the doctor immediately if any of them appear.
- Advise patient to avoid sudden position changes if orthostatic hypotension is a problem.

Biological response modifiers

aldesleukin

epoetin alfa

filgrastim

interferon alfa-2a, recombinant

interferon alfa-2b, recombinant

interferon alfa-n3

sargramostim

Biological response modifiers are products of recombinant DNA technology. All agents in this new drug class are synthetic versions of naturally occurring growth factors or immunomodulators.

Pharmacology

Biological response modifiers produce their effects in varying ways. By mimicking natural erythropoietin, epoetin alfa stimulates the rate of RBC production in the bone marrow. The glycoproteins filgrastim and sargramostim stimulate granulocyte (neutrophil) proliferation and differentiation. Sargramostim also promotes macrophage survival, differentiation, and production. The interleukin-2 derivative aldesleukin exhibits antitumor activity by an unknown mechanism. The recombinant interferons may exert direct antiproliferative action against tumor cells or viral cells. Interferon alfa-n3, a human leukocyte derivative, attaches to viral membrane receptors and causes cellular changes.

Clinical indications and actions

Aldesleukin is used to treat metastatic renal cell carcinoma. Epoetin alfa is used primarily to treat anemia caused by end-stage renal disease. Because of their hematopoietic effects, filgrastim and sargramostim are prescribed as adjunctive therapy for certain types of cancer. The recombinant interferons are used primarily to treat hairy-cell leukemia, acquired immunodeficiency syndrome (AIDS)-related Kaposi's sarcoma, and other cancers. Interferon alfa-n3 is used to treat condylomata acuminata. For more information, see the individual drug entries in this chapter.

Overview of adverse reactions

Aldesleukin, epoetin alfa, filgrastim, and sargramostim may cause adverse hematologic reactions, including blood dyscrasias. However, adverse cardiopulmonary reactions and electrolyte imbalances are more common with aldesleukin. Hypertension is the most common adverse reaction to epoetin alfa; bone pain, to filgrastim; and GI disturbances, to sargramostim. All interferons can produce adverse CNS and GI reactions. Recombinant interferons also are likely to cause adverse cardiovascular reactions.

Special considerations

- Perform standard hematologic tests before and during therapy to monitor for adverse hematologic reactions.
- Prepare and administer the prescribed biological response modifier precisely according to the facility's protocol and manufacturer's instructions.
- Take infection control measures, bleeding precautions, and energy conservation measures, as needed, for a patient who develops blood dyscrasias.
- Monitor for adverse CNS reactions and take safety precautions, as needed.
- Assess for adverse GI reactions; administer an antiemetic or other GI drug, if needed.

- Monitor blood pressure, ECG, hepatic and renal function studies, and serum electrolyte, BUN, and other levels as required by the specific drug.

Information for the patient
- Inform patient that aldesleukin or interferons can cause flulike symptoms, which usually resolve as therapy continues.
- Teach patient to recognize and report serious adverse reactions, such as arrhythmias and anaphylaxis.
- Teach patient to avoid persons with active infections, to take bleeding precautions, and to stagger activities and rest frequently.
- Stress the importance of returning for follow-up tests, as prescribed.
- Instruct patient how to prepare and self-administer the prescribed drug, if appropriate.

aldesleukin (interleukin-2, IL-2)
Proleukin
Pregnancy risk category: C

How supplied

Injection: 22 million IU/vial

Indications, route, and dosage

Metastatic renal cell carcinoma
Adults: 600,000 IU/kg (0.037 mg/kg) I.V. q 8 hours for 5 days (a total of 14 doses). After a 9-day rest, repeat the sequence for another 14 doses. Repeat courses may be administered after a rest period of at least 7 weeks after discharge.

Pharmacodynamics

Aldesleukin is a lymphokine, a highly purified immuno-regulatory protein synthesized using genetically engineered *Escherichia coli.* The drug produced is similar to human interleukin-2 (IL-2). It enhances lymphocyte mitogenesis, stimulates long-term growth of IL-2–dependent cell lines,

---

enhances lymphocyte cytotoxicity, induces both lympho-kine-activated and natural killer cell activity, and induces the production of interferon gamma.

Pharmacokinetics

Absorption: Aldesleukin is administered I.V.

Distribution: Peak serum levels are proportional to the dose. About 30% of drug rapidly distributes to the plasma; the balance is rapidly distributed to the liver, kidneys, and lungs. Initial studies indicate that the distribution half-life is about 13 minutes after a 5-minute I.V. infusion.

Metabolism: Aldesleukin is metabolized to amino acids within the cells lining the proximal convoluted tubules.

Excretion: Aldesleukin is excreted through the kidneys by peritubular extraction and glomerular filtration. Peritubular extraction ensures drug clearance as renal function diminishes and serum creatinine level rises. Elimination half-life is about 85 minutes.

Contraindications and precautions

Aldesleukin is contraindicated in patients with hypersensitivity to the drug or any of its components; the drug contains sodium dodecyl sulfate as a solubilizing agent. Aldesleukin is also contraindicated in patients who have received organ allografts (because it may increase the risk of allograft rejection in transplant recipients) and in patients with abnormal results on cardiac (thallium) stress tests or pulmonary function tests. Do not use unless the patient has had definitive tests documenting normal cardiac and pulmonary function.

Use with extreme caution in patients with normal test results if they have a history of cardiac or pulmonary disease. Also use cautiously in patients with a history of seizure disorders because the drug may cause seizures.

Retreatment is contraindicated in patients who experienced any of these toxicities from the drug: pericardial tamponade; abnormal cardiac rhythms that were uncontrolled or unresponsive to intervention; sustained ventricular tachycardia (five beats or more); chest pain accompanied by ECG changes, indicating MI or angina pectoris; renal dysfunction requiring dialysis for at least 72 hours; coma or toxic psychosis lasting at least 48 hours; seizures that were repetitive

---

or difficult to control; ischemia or perforation of the bowel; and GI bleeding requiring surgery.

Use cautiously and with close clinical monitoring because severe adverse effects generally accompany therapy at the recommended dosage. This drug should be used only in a hospital setting under the direction of a doctor experienced in the use of cancer chemotherapeutic drugs. An intensive care facility and specialists skilled in intensive care or cardiopulmonary medicine must be available.

Aldesleukin has also been associated with capillary leak syndrome (CLS), a condition that results from loss of vascular tone, which allows plasma proteins and fluids to escape into the extravascular space. Mean arterial blood pressure begins to drop within 2 to 12 hours of treatment. Edema and effusions may be severe, and death can result from hypoperfusion of major organs. Other conditions that accompany CLS include cardiac arrhythmias, MI, angina, mental status changes, renal insufficiency, respiratory distress or failure, and GI bleeding or infarction.

Interactions

Patients receiving antihypertensive drugs may be at increased risk for hypotension. Concomitant use with corticosteroids may decrease antitumor effectiveness of aldesleukin.

Aldesleukin may enhance the toxicity of hepatotoxic, nephrotoxic, cardiotoxic, or myelotoxic drugs. Because aldesleukin can alter CNS function, use cautiously with psychotropic drugs.

Effects on diagnostic tests

No direct laboratory test interference has been reported. Toxic effects of the drug may be reflected in abnormal hepatic, renal, and thyroid function tests; abnormal serum electrolyte levels; or abnormal cardiac or pulmonary function test results.

Adverse reactions

CNS: mental status changes, dizziness, sensory dysfunction, special senses disorders, syncope, motor dysfunction, headache, *coma.*

CV: hypotension, sinus tachycardia, *arrhythmias,* bradycardia, *premature ventricular contractions,* premature atrial contractions, *myocardial ischemia, MI, CHF, cardiac arrest, myocarditis, endocarditis, CVA,* pericardial effusion, thrombosis.

DERM: pruritus, erythema, rash, dryness, *exfoliative dermatitis,* purpura, alopecia, petechiae.

GI: nausea, vomiting, diarrhea, stomatitis, anorexia, *GI bleeding,* dyspepsia, constipation, abdominal pain.

GU: oliguria, *anuria,* proteinuria, hematuria, dysuria, urine retention, urinary frequency, urinary tract infection.

HEMA: anemia, thrombocytopenia, *leukopenia,* coagulation disorders, leukocytosis, eosinophilia.

Respiratory: *pulmonary congestion,* dyspnea, *pulmonary edema, respiratory failure, pleural effusion, apnea, pneumothorax,* tachypnea.

Other: jaundice; ascites; hepatomegaly; elevated bilirubin, BUN, serum creatinine, transaminase, and alkaline phosphatase levels; hypomagnesemia; acidosis; hypocalcemia; hypophosphatemia; hypokalemia; hyperuricemia; hypoalbuminemia; hypoproteinemia; hyponatremia; hyperkalemia; arthralgia; myalgia; fever; chills; chest or back pain; fatigue; weakness; malaise; edema; infections at the catheter tip or injection site; phlebitis; sepsis; weight gain; weight loss, conjunctivitis.

Overdose and treatment

Administration of high doses of aldesleukin will produce rapid onset of expected adverse reactions, including cardiac, renal, and hepatic toxicity.

Drug toxicity is dose-related. Treatment is supportive. Because aldesleukin's serum half-life is short, discontinuing the drug may ameliorate many of the adverse effects. Dexamethasone may decrease drug's toxicity but may also impair effectiveness.

Special considerations

• Perform standard hematologic tests, including CBC, differential, and platelet counts; serum electrolytes; and renal and hepatic function tests before therapy. Also obtain chest X-ray. Repeat daily during drug administration.

- Aldesleukin is associated with impaired neutrophil function, which can lead to disseminated infection. Many studies have employed prophylactic antibiotic therapy with oxacillin, nafcillin, ciprofloxacin, or vancomycin to counter this effect. Monitor for infection. Patients with bacterial infections should be treated before therapy with aldesleukin.
- Discontinue drug if patient develops moderate to severe lethargy or somnolence because continued administration can result in coma.
- Patients should be neurologically stable with no evidence of CNS metastases on computed tomography scan. Aldesleukin may exacerbate symptoms in patients with unrecognized or undiagnosed CNS metastases.
- Renal and hepatic impairment occur during treatment. Avoid administering other hepatotoxic or nephrotoxic drugs because toxicity may be additive. Also be prepared to adjust dosage of other drugs to compensate for this impairment. Dosage modification because of toxicity is usually accomplished by holding a dose or interrupting therapy rather than by reducing the dose to be administered.
- Severe anemia or thrombocytopenia may occur. Transfusion of packed RBCs or platelets may be necessary.
- Treat CLS with careful monitoring of fluid status, pulse, mental status, urine output, and organ perfusion. Central venous pressure monitoring is necessary.
- Because fluid management or administration of pressor agents may be essential to treat CLS, use cautiously in patients who require large volumes of fluid (such as patients with hypercalcemia).
- To avoid altering the drug's pharmacologic properties, reconstitute and dilute carefully, and follow manufacturer's recommendations. Do not mix with other drugs or albumin.
- Reconstitute a vial containing 22 million IU (1.3 mg) with 1.2 ml sterile water for injection. Do not use bacteriostatic water or 0.9% sodium chloride injection because these diluents cause increased aggregation of drug. Direct the stream at the sides of the vial and gently swirl to reconstitute. Do not shake.

---

*Canada only   †Off-label use   Italicized adverse reactions are life-threatening.

- The reconstituted solution will have a concentration of 18 million IU (1.1 mg)/ml. The reconstituted drug should be particle-free and colorless to slightly yellow.
- Add the correct dose of reconstituted drug to 50 ml of dextrose 5% in water and infuse over 15 minutes. Do not use an in-line filter. Plastic infusion bags are preferred because they provided consistent drug delivery in early clinical trials.
- Vials are for single use only and contain no preservative. Discard unused drug.
- Powder for injection or reconstituted solutions must be stored in the refrigerator. After reconstitution and dilution, drug must be administered within 48 hours. Be sure that solutions are returned to room temperature before administering drug to patient.
- Preliminary studies indicate that more than 75% of patients develop nonneutralizing antibodies to aldesleukin when treated with the every-8-hour dosing regimen. Fewer than 1% develop neutralizing antibodies. The clinical significance of this finding is not yet known.
- Aldesleukin has been investigated for treatment of various cancers, including Kaposi's sarcoma, metastatic melanoma, colorectal cancer, and non-Hodgkin's lymphoma.

Information for the patient
Make sure patient understands the serious toxicity that accompanies this drug. Adverse effects are expected with normal doses, and serious toxicity may occur despite close clinical monitoring.

epoetin alfa (erythropoietin)
Epogen, Procrit
Pregnancy risk category: C

How supplied
Injection: 2,000 units, 3,000 units, 4,000 units, 10,000 units

Indications, route, and dosage

Anemia associated with chronic renal failure

Adults: Initiate therapy at 50 to 100 units/kg three times weekly. Patients receiving dialysis should receive the drug I.V.; chronic renal failure patients not on dialysis may receive the drug S.C. or I.V.

Reduce dosage when the target hematocrit level is reached, or if the hematocrit rises more than 4 points within any 2-week period. Increase the dosage if the hematocrit level doesn't rise by 5 to 6 points after 8 weeks of therapy and the target range of 30% to 33% has not been reached.

Individualize the dosage for maintenance. Usually, the dosage is changed by 25 units/kg three times weekly.

Anemia related to zidovudine therapy in patients infected with human immunodeficiency virus (HIV)

Adults: Before therapy, determine endogenous serum erythropoietin levels. Patients with levels of 500 milliunits/ml or more are unlikely to respond to therapy. Initial dose for patients with levels of 500 milliunits/ml or less who are receiving 4,200 mg or less zidovudine weekly is 100 units/kg I.V. or S.C. three times weekly for 8 weeks. If response is inadequate after 8 weeks, increase dose by increments of 50 to 100 units/kg three times weekly and reevaluate response q 4 to 8 weeks. Individualize maintenance dose to maintain response, which may be influenced by zidovudine dose, infection, or inflammation.

Pharmacodynamics

Epoetin alfa is a glycoprotein consisting of 165 amino acids synthesized using recombinant DNA technology. It mimics naturally occurring erythropoietin, which is produced by the kidney. It stimulates the division and differentiation of cells within bone marrow to produce RBCs.

Pharmacokinetics

Absorption: Epoetin alfa may be given S.C. or I.V. After S.C. administration, peak serum levels occur within 5 to 24 hours.

Distribution: Information not available.

Metabolism: Information not available.

Excretion: Information not available.

Contraindications and precautions

Epoetin alfa is contraindicated in patients hypersensitive to mammalian cell-derived products or to human albumin. It is also contraindicated in patients with uncontrolled hypertension.

Interactions

None reported.

Effects on diagnostic tests

Moderate increases in BUN, uric acid, creatinine, phosphorus, and potassium levels have been reported.

Adverse reactions

CNS: headache.
CV: hypertension, clots at I.V. infusion site.
GI: nausea, diarrhea, vomiting.
Other: arthralgia, seizures.
   Note: Discontinue drug if the hematocrit level rises beyond target range of 30% to 33%.

Overdose and treatment

Maximum safe dose has not been established. Doses up to 1,500 units/kg have been administered three times weekly for 3 weeks without direct toxic effects.
   The drug can cause polycythemia; phlebotomy may be used to bring hematocrit within appropriate levels.

Special considerations

• Hematocrit level should be monitored at least twice weekly during the initiation of therapy and during any dosage adjustment. An interval of 2 to 6 weeks may elapse before a dosage change is reflected in the hematocrit level. The rapid rise in hematocrit can cause loss of blood pressure control. Reduce dosage so that the hematocrit doesn't increase by more than 4 points within any 2-week period. Monitor blood pressure as well. Epoetin alfa may have to be temporarily withheld until blood pressure is controlled.

- At the start of therapy, patients should avoid hazardous activities, such as driving or operating heavy machinery, because of a higher potential for seizures.
- Patients who are receiving dialysis may require increased anticoagulation with heparin.
- For HIV-infected patients treated with zidovudine, measure the hematocrit level once weekly until stabilized and then periodically.
- If patient fails to respond to epoetin alfa therapy, consider the following possible causes: vitamin deficiency, iron deficiency, underlying infection, occult blood loss, underlying hematologic disease, hemolysis, aluminum intoxication, osteitis fibrosa cystica, or increased dosage of zidovudine.
- Most patients eventually require supplemental iron therapy. Before and during therapy, monitor patient's iron stores, including serum ferritin and transferrin saturation.
- Routine monitoring of CBC with differential and platelet counts is recommended.

Information for the patient
- Explain the importance of regularly monitoring blood pressure in light of potential drug effects.
- Advise patient to adhere to dietary restrictions during therapy. Patient should understand that epoetin alfa will not influence the disease process.

filgrastim (granulocyte colony stimulating factor, G-CSF)
Neupogen
Pregnancy risk category: C

How supplied

Injection: 300 mcg/ml in 1-ml, 1.6-ml single-dose vials

Indications, route, and dosage

To decrease incidence of infection after cancer chemotherapy for nonmyeloid malignancies
Adults: Initially, 5 mcg/kg S.C. or I.V. as a single daily dose; may increase dose incrementally by 5 mcg/kg for each

---

course of chemotherapy according to duration and severity of absolute neutrophil count (ANC) nadir. Do not administer earlier than 24 hours after or within 24 hours before chemotherapy begins.

Filgrastim should be given daily for up to 2 weeks until ANC nadir reaches 10,000/mm³ after the anticipated nadir. Duration of treatment depends on the myelosuppressive potential of the chemotherapy used. Discontinue if ANC nadir surpasses 10,000/mm³.

Pharmacodynamics

Filgrastim is a naturally occurring cytokine glycoprotein that stimulates proliferation, differentiation, and functional activity of neutrophils, causing a rapid rise in WBC counts within 2 to 3 days in patients with normal bone marrow function or 7 to 14 days in patients with bone marrow suppression. Blood counts usually return to pretreatment levels within 1 week after therapy ends.

Pharmacokinetics

Absorption: After S.C. bolus dose, blood levels suggest rapid absorption, with peak levels in 4 to 5 hours.
Distribution: Unknown.
Metabolism: Unknown.
Excretion: Unknown.

Contraindications and precautions

Filgrastim is contraindicated in patients with hypersensitivity to products derived from *Escherichia coli*. Avoid use in patients with cancers with myeloid characteristics because filgrastim may act as a growth factor for any tumor.

Interactions

No evidence of drug interactions exists.

Effects on diagnostic tests

WBC counts may be increased to 100,000/mm³ or more. Transient increases in neutrophils, as well as reversible elevations in uric acid, LDH, and alkaline phosphatase levels, have been reported. Transient decreases in blood pressure and increases in serum creatinine, AST (formerly SGOT), and ALT (formerly SGPT) levels have also been reported.

Adverse reactions

CNS: skeletal pain, fatigue, headache, generalized weakness.
CV: chest pain, *arrhythmia, MI.*
DERM: alopecia, skin rash.
GI: nausea, vomiting, diarrhea, anorexia, constipation.
Respiratory: dyspnea, cough.
Other: stomatitis, neutropenic fever, mucositis, fever, sore throat, unspecified pain, splenomegaly.

Overdose and treatment

Maximum tolerated dose has not been determined. There have been no reports of overdose.

Special considerations

- Store in refrigerator; do not freeze. Avoid shaking. Before injection, allow to reach room temperature for a maximum of 6 hours. Discard after 6 hours. Use only one dose per vial; do not reenter the vial.
- Obtain CBC and platelet counts before therapy and twice weekly during therapy.
- Filgrastim is not compatible with 0.9% sodium chloride solution.
- Regular monitoring of hematocrit level and platelet count is recommended.
- Adult respiratory distress syndrome may occur in septic patients because of the influx of neutrophils at the site of inflammation.
- MI and arrhythmias have occurred; closely monitor patients with preexisting cardiac conditions.
- Bone pain is the most frequent adverse reaction and may be controlled with nonnarcotic analgesics if mild to moderate; if severe, treatment with narcotic analgesics may be necessary.

Information for the patient
- Review the patient-information section of the package insert with patient. Thorough instruction is essential if home use is prescribed.

- When drug can be safely and effectively self-administered, instruct patient in proper dosage and administration techniques.
- Manufacturer has reimbursement hot line to answer questions about insurance reimbursement procedures. The hot line operates from Monday through Friday 9 a.m. to 5 p.m. Eastern Standard Time: 1-800-272-9376; in Washington, D.C.: 1-202-637-6698.

interferon alfa-2a, recombinant
Roferon-A

interferon alfa-2b, recombinant
Intron A

Pregnancy risk category: C

How supplied

Roferon A
3 million IU/vial; 18 million IU/multiple-dose vial for injection; 36 million IU/vial for injection
Intron A
3 million IU/vial, 5 million IU/vial, 10 million IU/vial, 25 million IU/vial, 50 million IU/vial with diluent for injection

Indications, route, and dosage

Hairy-cell leukemia
Alfa-2a
Adults: For induction, give 3 million units S.C. or I.M. daily for 16 to 24 weeks. For maintenance, 3 million units S.C. or I.M. three times weekly.
Alfa-2b
Adults: 2 million units/m² I.M. or S.C. three times weekly (for both induction and maintenance).
Condylomata acuminata
Alfa-2b
Adults: 1 million units per lesion, intralesionally, three times a week for 3 weeks.

Kaposi's sarcoma
Alfa-2a
Adults: Induction therapy is 36 million IU S.C. or I.M. daily for 10 to 12 weeks; maintenance dose is 36 million IU three times weekly.
Alfa-2b
Adults: 30 million IU/m^2 S.C. or I.M. three times weekly. Maintain this dose unless the disease progresses rapidly or intolerance occurs.
Chronic hepatitis C
Alfa-2b
Adults: 3 million IU S.C. or I.M. three times weekly. If response occurs, continue therapy for 6 months. If no response by 16 weeks, discontinue therapy.

Pharmacodynamics

Interferon alfa is a sterile protein product produced by recombinant DNA techniques applied to genetically engineered *Escherichia coli*. The interferons are naturally occurring small protein molecules produced and secreted by cells in response to viral infections or synthetic and biological inducers. They act through a direct antiproliferative action against tumor or viral cells to inhibit replication and modulation of host immune response by enhancing the phagocytic activity of macrophages and augmenting the specific cytotoxicity of lymphocytes for target cells.

Pharmacokinetics

Absorption: More than 80% of dose is absorbed after I.M. or S.C. injection.
Distribution: Not applicable.
Metabolism: Interferon alfa appears to be metabolized in the liver and kidney.
Excretion: Interferon alfa is reabsorbed from glomerular filtrate with minor biliary elimination.

Contraindications and precautions

Interferons are contraindicated in patients with hypersensitivity to them or to any components of the product.

Interferons should be used cautiously in patients with severe hepatic or renal function impairment, seizure disor-

---

ders, compromised CNS function, cardiac disease, or myelo-suppression because they may worsen these conditions.

Interactions

When used concomitantly with CNS depressants, interferons may enhance their CNS effects.

Concurrent use of interfron alfa with a live virus vaccine may potentiate replication of vaccine virus, increase adverse effects, and decrease patient's antibody response.

Bone marrow depressant effects may be increased when interferon alfa is used with blood dyscrasia–causing medications, bone marrow depressant therapy, or radiation therapy. Dosage reduction may be required. Interferon may substantially increase the half-life of methylxanthines (including theophylline and aminophylline), perhaps by interfering with cytochrome P-450 drug metabolizing enzymes.

Effects on diagnostic tests

Interferon therapy may cause mild and transient alterations of blood pressure (hypotension is likely). Interferons may decrease hemoglobin and hematocrit levels, and WBC, platelet, and neutrophil counts (dose-related; recovery occurs within several days or weeks after withdrawal of interferon). Interferons may increase prothrombin time and partial thromboplastin time (dose-related); ALT (formerly SGPT), AST (formerly SGOT), LDH, and alkaline phosphatase levels (dose-related; reversible on withdrawal of interferon); and serum calcium, serum phosphorus, and fasting blood glucose levels.

Adverse reactions

CNS: dizziness, confusion, paresthesia, numbness, lethargy, depression, nervousness, difficulty in thinking or concentrating, trouble sleeping, sedation, apathy, anxiety, irritability, fatigue.
CV: hypotension, chest pain, *arrhythmias*, palpitations, *CHF,* syncope, hypertension, edema.
DERM: rash, dryness, pruritus, partial alopecia, urticaria.
GI: anorexia, nausea, diarrhea, vomiting, abdominal fullness, taste alteration.
GU: transient impotence.

---

*Canada only   †Off-label use   Italicized adverse reactions are life-threatening.

HEMA: *leukopenia,* mild thrombocytopenia.
Other: pharyngitis, sneezing, dry or inflamed oropharynx, flulike symptoms (fever, headache, chills, muscle aches).

Overdose and treatment

No information available.

Special considerations

- When preparing interferons for injection, take special precautions because of their potential for carcinogenicity and mutagenicity. Use of a biological safety cabinet is recommended. Do not shake vials.
- Administer by S.C. route in patients whose platelet count is below 50,000/mm³.
- Different brands of interferons may not be therapeutically interchangeable.
- Almost all patients experience flulike symptoms at the beginning of therapy. These effects tend to diminish with continued therapy.
- Patient should be well hydrated, especially during initial stages of treatment. Premedicate with acetaminophen to minimize flulike symptoms.
- Dosage reduction may be needed if headache persists. Hypotension may result from fluid depletion and may require supportive treatment.
- Administration at bedtime minimizes inconvenience of fatigue.
- Monitor blood pressure; BUN; hematocrit; platelet count; total and differential WBC count; ECG; and ALT, AST, LDH, alkaline phosphatase, serum bilirubin, creatinine, and uric acid levels.
- Monitor for CNS adverse reactions, such as decreased mental status and dizziness. Periodic neuropsychiatric monitoring is recommended.
- Take these special precautions for patients who develop thrombocytopenia: Exercise extreme care in performing invasive procedures; inspect injection site and skin frequently for signs of bruising; limit frequency of I.M. injections; test urine, emesis fluid, stool, and secretions for occult blood.

- When using interferon alfa-2b for condylomata acuminata by intralesional injection, use only the 10 million-unit vial reconstituted with 1 ml of diluent. Using other strengths or more diluent would produce a hypertonic solution. For administration, use a 25G to 30G needle and a tuberculin syringe. Up to five lesions may be treated simultaneously.
- The following indications are not included in U.S. labeling, but interferons may be used for these applications: chronic myelocytic leukemia; treatment of renal carcinoma, superficial bladder carcinoma; treatment of non-Hodgkin's lymphomas, especially nodular, poorly differentiated types; malignant melanoma; multiple myeloma; mycosis fungoides; papillomas; and laryngeal papillomatosis (interferon alfa-2b).

Information for the patient

- Review patient instruction sheet if patient is to self-administer the drug to ensure patient understanding of when and how to take medication. Stress importance of drinking extra fluids to prevent hypotension from fluid loss.
- Instruct patient in proper oral hygiene during treatment, because the bone marrow depressant effects of interferons may result in increased incidence of microbial infection, delayed healing, and gingival bleeding. A decrease in salivary flow may also occur.
- Advise patient not to take a missed dose or to double the next dose, but to call for further instructions.
- If patient is to self-administer drug, teach patient to prepare injection, how to use disposable syringe, proper administration technique, and stability of drug.
- Store drug in refrigerator; keep from freezing.
- Caution patient against driving or performing tasks requiring alertness until response to medication is known.
- Advise patient to avoid use of aspirin and excessive use of alcohol because they may increase the risk of GI bleeding.
- Advise patient to seek medical approval before taking nonprescription medications for colds, coughs, allergies, and similar disorders; explain that interferons commonly cause flulike symptoms and patient may need to take acetaminophen before each dose.

- Emphasize need to follow instructions about taking and recording temperature, and how and when to take acetaminophen.
- Caution patient to avoid immunizations and contact with persons who have taken oral polio vaccine. Because the body's resistance may be compromised, infection may occur.
- Tell patient drug may cause temporary loss of some hair. Normal hair growth should return when drug is withdrawn.

Geriatric use
Neurotoxicity and cardiotoxicity are more common in elderly patients, especially those with underlying CNS or cardiac impairment.

interferon alfa-n3
Alferon N
Pregnancy risk category: C

How supplied
Injection: 5 million IU/ml, in 1-ml vials

Indications, route, and dosage
Indications and dosage may vary. Check literature for current protocol.
Condylomata acuminata
Adults: 0.5 ml (250,000 IU) per wart injected into the base of each wart twice weekly for up to 8 weeks. For large warts, inject at several points around the periphery of the wart using a total dose of 0.5 ml per wart. Maximum dose for each treatment is 0.5 ml per wart. Use a 30G needle.

Pharmacodynamics
The interferons are naturally occurring small-protein molecules produced and secreted by cells in response to viral infections and biological inducers. They bind to specific membrane receptors on cell surfaces to initiate a series of events that include induction of protein synthesis, which is

then followed by various cellular responses (inhibition of virus replication, suppression of cell proliferation, immuno-modulation, enhanced phagocytosis, augmentation of lym-phocytic cytotoxicity, and enhancement of human leukocyte antigen expression). The exact mechanism of action is not known.

Pharmacokinetics

Absorption: After intralesional injection, plasma concentra-tions are below detectable levels, but systemic effects indicate that some systemic absorption does occur.
Distribution: Unknown.
Metabolism: Unknown.
Excretion: Unknown.

Contraindications and precautions

Contraindicated in patients with hypersensitivity to human interferon alfa or to any component of the injection and in patients who have anaphylactic sensitivity to mouse immu-noglobulin G, egg protein, or neomycin. Use with caution in patients with debilitating medical conditions, such as cardiac disease, severe pulmonary disease, diabetes mellitus with ketoacidosis, coagulation disorders, seizure disorders, or se-vere myelosuppression because the drug may worsen these conditions.

Interactions

None reported.

Effects on diagnostic tests

Decreases in WBC counts have been reported. The following laboratory values were abnormal in cancer patients: hemo-globin, WBC count, platelet count, gamma-glutamyl trans-ferase, AST (formerly SGOT) level, alkaline phosphatase level, and total bilirubin level.

Adverse reactions

CNS: dizziness, light-headedness, insomnia, sleepiness, fatigue, malaise, headache, depression.
CV: hypotension, chest pain.

DERM: generalized pruritus, photosensitivity.
EENT: nose and sinus drainage, epistaxis, pharyngitis, blurred vision, ocular rotation pain.
GI: nausea, vomiting, diarrhea, constipation, dyspepsia, heartburn, anorexia, stomatitis, mucositis.
Other: flulike syndrome, fever, chills, sweating, vasovagal reaction, myalgia, arthralgia, soreness at injection site, back pain, left groin lymph node swelling.

Overdose and treatment

No information available.

Special considerations

- Different brands of interferons may not be therapeutically interchangeable.
- Almost all patients experience flulike symptoms, which diminish with continued therapy.
- Genital warts usually begin to disappear after several weeks of therapy, but treatment should continue for the full 8 weeks. In patients who experience partial resolution during treatment, further resolution occurs after treatment ends. Of those patients who experienced complete resolution, half had complete resolution by the end of treatment; the rest within 3 months posttreatment.
- Do not administer further treatment for 3 months after first course of therapy unless warts enlarge or new warts appear.
- Flulike symptoms are relieved by acetaminophen.
- Interferon alfa-n3 is manufactured from pooled units of human WBCs induced by incomplete infection with an avian virus. Donors are screened to minimize risk of human immunodeficiency virus (HIV) and hepatitis B. There are no reported incidents of HIV or hepatitis B transmission.
- Store in refrigerator; do not freeze. Do not shake.
- Use 30G needle to administer.
- Interferon alfa-n3 has been used for the following unlabeled indications: hairy-cell leukemia, bladder tumors, carcinoid tumors, chronic myelogenous leukemia, cutaneous T-cell lymphoma, essential thrombocythemia, non-Hodgkin's lymphoma (low grade), cervical cancer, chronic lym-

---

*Canada only   †Off-label use   Italicized adverse reactions are life-threatening.

phocytic leukemia, acute leukemias, osteosarcoma, AIDS-related Kaposi's sarcoma, malignant gliomas, melanoma, multiple myeloma, nasopharyngeal sarcoma, ovarian cancer, renal carcinoma, cutaneous warts, cytomegaloviruses, herpes keratoconjunctivitis, herpes simplex, papillomaviruses, rhinoviruses, vaccinia virus, varicella zoster, viral hepatitis B, and chronic hepatitis C.

Information for the patient
- Advise patient of risks and benefits of therapy.
- Tell patient to watch for signs of anaphylaxis—local or generalized hives, tightness of the chest, wheezing, and dizziness or weakness—and to call doctor if they develop.

sargramostim (granulocyte macrophage-colony stimulating factor, GM-CSF)
Leukine, Prokine

Pregnancy risk category: C

How supplied

Injection (preservative-free): 250 mcg, 500 mcg (as lyophilized powder) in single-dose vials

Indications, route, and dosage

Acceleration of hematopoietic reconstitution after autologous bone marrow transplantation in patients with non-Hodgkin's lymphoma, acute lymphoblastic leukemia, or Hodgkin's disease undergoing autologous bone marrow transplantation (BMT)
Adults: 250 mcg/m² daily for 21 consecutive days given as a 2-hour I.V. infusion daily beginning 2 to 4 hours after BMT. Do not administer within 24 hours of last dose of chemotherapy or within 12 hours after the last dose of radiotherapy because of the potential sensitivity of rapidly dividing progenitor cells to cytotoxic chemotherapeutic or radiologic therapies.

 Reduce dosage by half or temporarily discontinue if severe adverse reactions occur. Therapy may be resumed when reaction abates. If blast cells appear or increase to 10% or more of the WBC count or if progression of the underlying disease occurs, discontinue therapy. If absolute neutrophil count is above 20,000 cells/mm³ or if WBC counts are above 50,000 cells/mm³, therapy should be discontinued temporarily or the dose reduced by half.

Bone marrow transplantation failure or engraftment delay
Adults: 250 mcg/m² daily for 14 days as a 2-hour I.V. infusion. The same course may be repeated after 7 days off therapy if engraftment has not occurred. A third course of 500 mcg/m² daily for 14 days may be given after another 7 days off therapy if engraftment has not occurred.

Pharmacodynamics

Sargramostim is a 127-amino acid glycoprotein manufactured by recombinant DNA technology in a yeast expression system. It differs from natural human GM-CSF by substitution of leucine for arginine at position 23. The carbohydrate moiety may also be different. Sargramostim induces cellular responses by binding to specific receptors on cell surfaces of target cells. Blood counts return to normal or baseline levels within 3 to 7 days after stopping treatment.

Pharmacokinetics

Absorption: Blood levels are detected within 5 minutes after I.V. administration; peak levels, within 2 hours.
Distribution: Bound to specific receptors on target cells.
Metabolism: Undetermined.
Excretion: Unknown.

Contraindications and precautions

Sargramostim is contraindicated in patients with excessive leukemic myeloid blasts in bone marrow or peripheral blood and in patients with known hypersensitivity to the drug, any of its components, or yeast-derived products. Use with caution in patients with preexisting cardiac disease, hypoxia, preexisting fluid retention, pulmonary infiltrates, CHF, or impaired renal or hepatic function because these conditions may be exacerbated.

Interactions

Lithium and corticosteroids should be used with caution because they may potentiate sargramostim's myeloproliferative effects.

Effects on diagnostic tests

No interference reported. Because hematopoiesis is stimulated, effects on CBC and differential blood counts will be observed.

Adverse reactions

CNS: malaise, asthenia.
CV: *blood dyscrasias,* hemorrhage.
DERM: alopecia, rash.
GI: nausea, vomiting, diarrhea, anorexia, GI hemorrhage, stomatitis, liver damage.
GU: urinary tract disorder, abnormal kidney function.
Respiratory: dyspnea.
Other: fever, edema, peripheral edema, *sepsis.*

Overdose and treatment

Doses up to 16 times the recommended dose have been administered with the following reversible adverse reactions: WBC counts up to 200,000/mm^3, dyspnea, malaise, nausea, fever, rash, sinus tachycardia, headache, and chills. The maximum dose that can be administered safely has yet to be determined. If overdose is suspected, monitor increase in WBC count and respiratory symptoms.

Special considerations

- Stimulation of marrow precursors may result in rapid rise of WBC count; biweekly monitoring of CBC with differential, including examination for blast cells, is recommended.
- Transient rashes and local injection site reactions may occur; no serious allergic or anaphylactic reactions have been reported.
- Sargramostim can act as a growth factor for any tumor type, particularly myeloid cancers.

- Sargramostim is effective in accelerating myeloid recovery in patients receiving bone marrow purged from monoclonal antibodies.
- The effect of sargramostim may be limited in patients who have received extensive radiotherapy to hematopoietic sites for treatment of primary disease in the abdomen or chest or have been exposed to multiple agents (alkylating agents, anthracycline antibiotics, antimetabolites) before autologous BMT.
- Refrigerate the sterile powder, the reconstituted solution, and the diluted solution for injection. Do not freeze or shake. Do not use after expiration date.
- To prepare, reconstitute the powder with 1 ml sterile water for injection. Do not reenter or reuse the single-dose vial. Discard any unused portion. Direct stream of sterile water against the side of the vial and gently swirl contents to minimize foaming. Avoid excessive or vigorous agitation or shaking. Dilute in 0.9% sodium chloride solution. If final concentration is below 10 mcg/ml, add 1% albumin (1 mg albumin/ml of sodium chloride) to the solution before you add sargramostim to prevent adherence to the I.V. container and tubing.
- Administer as soon as possible after admixture, as sargramostim has no preservative, and within 6 hours of reconstitution or dilution.
- Do not add other medications to the infusion solution without compatibility and stability data.
- Discard any unused solution after 6 hours.
- Refrigerate the sterile powder, the reconstituted solution, and the diluted solution for injection. Do not freeze or shake. Do not use after expiration date.
- Sargramostim has been used to increase WBC counts in patients with myelodysplastic syndromes and in AIDS patients receiving zidovudine; to decrease nadir of leukopenia secondary to myelosuppressive chemotherapy; to decrease myelosuppression in preleukemic patients; to correct neutropenia in aplastic anemia; and to decrease transplant-associated organ system damage, particularly of the liver and kidneys.

Information for the patient
Remind patient to avoid persons with infection.

Miscellaneous antineoplastics

altretamine	paclitaxel
asparaginase	prednisone
etoposide	teniposide
hydroxyurea	vinblastine sulfate
methylprednisolone	vincristine sulfate

The drugs in this chapter fall into a number of different classifications. Refer to the individual entry for specific information about that drug and its clinical use.

altretamine (hexamethylmelamine)
Hexalen, Hexastat*

Pregnancy risk category: D

How supplied

Capsules: 50 mg

Indications, route, and dosage

Palliative treatment of persistent or recurrent ovarian cancer after first-line therapy with cisplatin or alkylating agent combination
Single agent therapy
Women: 260 mg/m²/day P.O. in four divided doses (after meals and h.s.) for 14 to 21 consecutive days in a 28-day cycle.

Combination therapy

Women: 150 mg/m²/day P.O. in four divided doses (after meals and h.s.) administered on days 1 to 14 of a 28-day cycle. Used with cyclophosphamide and doxorubicin, with or without cisplatin.

Pharmacodynamics

The precise mechanism of action is unknown. Metabolism in the liver is required for cytotoxicity. Although it is structurally similar to the alkylating agent triethylenemelamine, altretamine and its metabolites have not demonstrated alkylating activity on in vitro tests.

Pharmacokinetics

Absorption: Altretamine is well absorbed from the GI tract after oral administration; however, rapid and extensive demethylation causes variations in plasma levels.

Distribution: Altretamine does not cross the blood-brain barrier to a significant extent. The drug and its metabolites show binding to plasma proteins.

Metabolism: Altretamine undergoes rapid and extensive demethylation in the liver.

Excretion: Metabolites are excreted primarily in the urine. A small amount is eliminated through the lungs in expired air; trace amounts are excreted in feces.

Contraindications and precautions

Altretamine is contraindicated in patients with known hypersensitivity to the drug and in patients with preexisting severe bone marrow depression or severe neurotoxicity.

Interactions

Concurrent administration of MAO inhibitors with altretamine may cause severe orthostatic hypotension. Concurrent use with cimetidine increases altretamine's half-life and the potential for toxicity because cimetidine inhibits microsomal drug metabolism.

Effects on diagnostic tests

Blood and urine uric acid concentrations may be increased; serum creatinine and BUN levels may be altered.

Adverse reactions

CNS: mild to moderate neurotoxicity, peripheral neuropathy, mood disorders, ataxia, dizziness, vertigo, consciousness disorders, fatigue, seizures.
GI: mild to severe dose-related nausea and vomiting, increased alkaline phosphatase level, anorexia.
HEMA: mild to *severe anemia*, leukopenia, *thrombocytopenia*.
Other: *hepatotoxicity*, skin rash, pruritus, alopecia.

Overdose and treatment

Clinical manifestations of overdose include myelosuppression and severe nausea and vomiting unresponsive to usual treatment. Symptoms are more likely to occur in patients receiving continuous high-dose daily altretamine. Neurotoxicity appears reversible and may be diminished by concurrent administration of pyridoxine.

Treatment is usually supportive and may include administration of antiemetics and transfusion of blood components.

Special considerations

- Unresponsive GI intolerance, WBC count below 2,000/mm^3 or granulocyte count below 1,000/mm^3, platelet count below 7,500/mm^3, and progressive neurotoxicity require temporary discontinuation for 14 days or more and a dosage reduction to 200 mg/m^2 daily when restarted.
- Monitor peripheral blood counts at least monthly and before each course of therapy.
- Premedication with antiemetics may decrease incidence or severity of nausea and vomiting.
- Tolerance to GI effects may develop after several weeks of therapy. If severity is uncontrolled with antiemetics, dosage reduction may be required.
- Perform neurologic examinations regularly during administration to check for neurotoxicity. Concomitant administration of 100 mg pyridoxine may diminish neurotoxicity.

Information for the patient
- Tell patient to call doctor if vomiting occurs shortly after the dose is taken.
- Emphasize importance of continuing to take medication despite occasional nausea and vomiting.
- Encourage fluid intake to increase urine output and facilitate uric acid excretion.
- Instruct patient to report any signs of neurotoxicity.
- Instruct patient to avoid exposure to persons with infections.

asparaginase
Elspar, Kidrolase

Pregnancy risk category: C

How supplied

Injection: 10,000-IU vials

Indications, route, and dosage

Indications and dosage may vary. Check current literature for recommended protocol.

Acute lymphocytic leukemia
Adults and children: When used alone, 200 IU/kg daily I.V. for 28 days. When used in combination with other chemotherapeutic drugs, dosage is highly individualized.

Pharmacodynamics

Asparaginase exerts its cytotoxic activity by inactivating the amino acid asparagine, which is required by tumor cells to synthesize proteins. Because the tumor cells cannot synthesize their own asparagine, protein synthesis and eventually synthesis of DNA and RNA are inhibited.

Pharmacokinetics

Absorption: Asparaginase is not absorbed across the GI tract after oral administration; therefore, the drug must be given I.V. or I.M.
Distribution: Asparaginase distributes primarily within the intravascular space, with detectable concentrations in the tho-

racic and cervical lymph. The drug crosses the blood-brain barrier to a minimal extent.

Metabolism: The metabolic fate of asparaginase is unclear; hepatic sequestration by the reticuloendothelial system may occur.

Excretion: The plasma elimination half-life, which is not related to dose, sex, age, or hepatic or renal function, ranges from 8 to 30 hours.

Contraindications and precautions

Asparaginase is contraindicated in patients with a history of anaphylactoid reactions to the drug or in patients with pancreatitis or a history of pancreatitis.

Asparaginase should be used cautiously in patients with impaired liver function, infections, or recent therapy with antineoplastic agents or radiation because of risk of increased adverse effects.

Interactions

Concomitant use of asparaginase with methotrexate decreases the effectiveness of methotrexate because asparaginase destroys the actively replicating cells that methotrexate requires for its cytotoxic action. Concomitant use of asparaginase and vincristine can cause additive neuropathy and disturbances of erythropoiesis. When asparaginase is used with prednisone, hyperglycemia may result from an additive effect on the pancreas.

Effects on diagnostic tests

Asparaginase therapy alters the results of thyroid function tests by decreasing concentrations of serum thyroxine-binding globulin.

Adverse reactions

CNS: lethargy, somnolence, headache, confusion, agitation, tremor.
DERM: rash, urticaria.
GI: vomiting (may last up to 24 hours), anorexia, nausea, cramps, weight loss, stomatitis.

GU: azotemia, *renal failure,* uric acid nephropathy, glycosuria, polyuria.
HEMA: hypofibrinogenemia and depression of other clotting
factors, *thrombocytopenia, leukopenia,* depression of serum
albumin.
Hepatic: elevated AST (formerly SGOT) and ALT (formerly
SGPT) levels, hepatotoxicity.
Metabolic: elevated alkaline phosphatase and bilirubin (direct
and indirect) levels; increase or decrease in total lipids; hyperglycemia; increased blood ammonia level.
Other: *hemorrhagic pancreatitis, anaphylaxis* (relatively common).
   Note: Drug should be discontinued at the first sign of renal failure or pancreatitis.

Overdose and treatment

Clinical manifestations of overdose include nausea and diarrhea.
   Treatment is generally supportive and includes administration of antiemetics and antidiarrheals.

Special considerations

- Reconstitute asparaginase for I.M. administration with
  2 ml unpreserved 0.9% sodium chloride solution or sterile
  water for injection.
- Do not use reconstituted drug if precipitate forms.
- I.M. injections should not contain more than 2 ml per injection. Multiple injections may be used for each dose.
- Reconstitute asparaginase for I.V. administration with 5
  ml of sterile water for injection or sodium chloride injection. Solution will be clear or slightly cloudy. May further
  dilute with sodium chloride injection or dextrose 5% in
  water and administer I.V. over 30 minutes. Filtration
  through a 5-micron in-line filter during administration
  will remove particulate matter that may develop on standing; filtration through a 0.22-micron filter will result in a
  loss of potency. Do not use if precipitate forms.
- Shake vial gently when reconstituting. Vigorous shaking
  will result in decreased potency.

- Refrigerate unopened dry powder. Reconstituted solution is stable for 6 hours at room temperature and 24 hours if refrigerated.
- Don't use as sole agent to induce remission unless combination therapy is inappropriate. Not recommended for maintenance therapy.
- Asparaginase should be administered in a hospital setting with close supervision.
- I.V. administration of asparaginase with or immediately before vincristine or prednisone may increase toxicity reactions.
- Conduct skin test before initial dose. Observe site for 1 hour. Erythema and wheal formation indicate a positive reaction.
- Risk of hypersensitivity increases with repeated doses. Patient may be desensitized, but this doesn't rule out risk of allergic reactions. Routine administration of 2-unit I.V. test dose may identify high-risk patients.
- Because of vomiting, patient may need parenteral fluids for 24 hours or until oral fluids are tolerated.
- Monitor CBC and bone marrow function. Bone marrow regeneration may take 5 to 6 weeks.
- Obtain frequent serum amylase determinations to check pancreatic status. If elevated, asparaginase should be discontinued.
- Tumor lysis can result in uric acid nephropathy. Prevent occurrence by increasing fluid intake. Allopurinol should be started before therapy begins.
- Watch for signs of bleeding, such as petechiae and melena.
- Monitor blood glucose and test urine before and during therapy. Watch for signs of hyperglycemia, such as glycosuria and polyuria.
- Keep epinephrine, diphenhydramine, and I.V. corticosteroids available for treatment of anaphylaxis.

Information for the patient
- Encourage adequate intake of fluids to increase urine output and facilitate uric acid excretion.
- Tell patient drowsiness may occur during therapy or for several weeks after treatment has ended. Tell patient to avoid hazardous activities requiring mental alertness.

etoposide (VP-16)
VePesid

Pregnancy risk category: D

How supplied

Injection: 100 mg/5 ml multiple-dose vials
Capsules: 50 mg

Indications, route, and dosage

Indications and dosage may vary. Check literature for current protocol.

Small-cell carcinoma of the lung

Adults: 70 mg/m²/day P.O. (rounded to the nearest 50 mg) for 4 days, or 100 mg/m² P.O. (rounded to the nearest 50 mg) daily for 5 days. Repeat q 3 to 4 weeks. Alternatively, 35 mg/m² I.V. daily for 4 days, or 50 mg/m² I.V. daily for 5 days. Repeat q 3 to 4 weeks.

Testicular cancer

Men: 50 to 100 mg/m² I.V. daily on days 1 to 5; or 100 mg/m²/day I.V. on days 1, 3, and 5 of a regimen repeated q 3 or 4 weeks.

Pharmacodynamics

Etoposide exerts its cytotoxic action by arresting cells in the metaphase portion of cell division. The drug also inhibits cells from entering mitosis and depresses DNA and RNA synthesis.

Pharmacokinetics

Absorption: Etoposide is only moderately absorbed across the GI tract after oral administration. The bioavailability ranges from 25% to 75%, with an average of 50% of the dose being absorbed.

Distribution: Etoposide distributes widely into body tissues; the highest concentrations are found in the liver, spleen, kidneys, healthy brain tissue, and brain tumor tissue. The drug crosses the blood-brain barrier to a limited and variable extent. Etoposide is approximately 94% bound to serum albumin.

Metabolism: Only a small portion of a dose of etoposide is metabolized. Metabolism occurs in the liver.

Excretion: Etoposide is excreted primarily in the urine as unchanged drug. A smaller portion of a dose is excreted in the feces. The plasma elimination of etoposide is described as biphasic, with an initial phase half-life of about $1/2$ to 2 hours and a terminal phase half-life of about $5 1/2$ to 11 hours.

Contraindications and precautions

Etoposide is contraindicated in patients with a history of hypersensitivity to the drug.

Interactions

Concomitant use of etoposide increases the cytotoxicity of cisplatin against certain tumors. The mechanism of this synergistic cytotoxic activity is unknown.

Effects on diagnostic tests

None reported.

Adverse reactions

CNS: headache, weakness, visual disturbances, peripheral neuropathy (especially if administered with other neurotoxic medications).

CV: hypotension from rapid infusion, palpitations, tachycardia.

GI: nausea and vomiting, anorexia, stomatitis.

HEMA: *bone marrow depression* (dose-limiting), *leukopenia, thrombocytopenia.* (*Note:* Drug should be discontinued if severe hematopoietic toxicity results.)

Local: infrequent phlebitis; pain at I.V. site.

Other: occasional fever, reversible alopecia, *anaphylaxis* (rare), generalized pain, chills, diaphoresis.

Overdose and treatment

Clinical manifestations of overdose include myelosuppression, nausea, and vomiting.

Treatment is usually supportive and includes transfusion of blood components, administration of antiemetics, and appropriate symptomatic therapy.

---

*Canada only   †Off-label use   Italicized adverse reactions are life-threatening.

Special considerations

- To prepare solution, dilute prescribed dose to a concentration of 0.2 to 0.4 mg/ml with 0.9% sodium chloride solution or dextrose 5% in water. Higher concentrations may crystallize. Discard solution if cloudy.
- Solutions diluted to 0.2 mg/ml are stable for 96 hours at room temperature in plastic or glass containers unprotected from light; solutions diluted to 0.4 mg/ml are stable for 48 hours under the same conditions.
- Administer infusion over 30 to 60 minutes to avoid hypotensive reactions.
- Treat extravasation with local injections of hyaluronidase, which aids in systemic reabsorption of etoposide.
- Pretreat the patient with antiemetics to reduce frequency and duration of nausea and vomiting.
- GI toxicity occurs more frequently after oral administration.
- At doses below 200 mg, extent of absorption after oral administration is not affected by food.
- Intrapleural and intrathecal administration of etoposide is contraindicated due to severe toxicity.
- Dosage reduction may be required for patients with impaired renal function.
- Capsules must be stored under refrigeration.
- Have diphenhydramine, hydrocortisone, epinephrine, and an airway available in case of an anaphylactic reaction.
- Monitor blood pressure before infusion and at 30-minute intervals during infusion. If systolic blood pressure falls below 90 mm Hg, stop infusion.
- Monitor CBC. Observe patient for signs of bone marrow depression.
- Because of the risk of serious adverse reactions in the infant, breast-feeding is not recommended.

Information for the patient

- Emphasize importance of continuing medication despite nausea and vomiting.
- Tell patient to call immediately if vomiting occurs shortly after dose is taken.
- Advise patient to avoid exposure to persons with infections.

- Tell patient not to receive immunizations during therapy with etoposide. Other members of the patient's household should also avoid immunizations during the same period.
- Tell patient to promptly report a sore throat, fever, or unusual bruising or bleeding.
- Reassure patient that hair should grow back after treatments ends.

Geriatric use
Elderly patients may be particularly susceptible to the hypotensive effects of etoposide.

hydroxyurea
Hydrea
Pregnancy risk category: C

How supplied

Capsules: 500 mg

Indications, route, and dosage

Indications and dosage may vary. Check current literature for recommended protocol.
Melanoma; chronic myelocytic leukemia; recurrent, metastatic, or inoperable ovarian cancer; squamous cell carcinoma of the head and neck; †polycythemia vera; †essential thrombocytosis
Adults: 60 to 80 mg/kg P.O. or 2,000 to 3,000 mg/m² P.O. as single dose q 3 days, or 20 to 30 mg/kg P.O. daily for a minimum of 6 weeks. Dosage is based on ideal body weight if patient is obese or has fluid retention.
†To increase hemoglobin F production in patients with sickle-cell trait
Adults: 7.5 to 40 mg P.O. daily; the median dose reported in some studies is 20 mg/kg.

Pharmacodynamics

The exact mechanism of hydroxyurea's cytotoxic action is unclear. Hydroxyurea inhibits DNA synthesis without interfering with RNA or protein synthesis. The drug may act as an antimetabolite, inhibiting the incorporation of thymidine into DNA, and may also damage DNA directly.

Pharmacokinetics

Absorption: Hydroxyurea is well absorbed after oral administration, with peak serum levels occurring 2 hours after a dose. Higher serum levels are achieved if the drug is given as a large single dose rather than in divided doses.
Distribution: Hydroxyurea crosses the blood-brain barrier.
Metabolism: Approximately 50% of an oral dose is degraded in the liver.
Excretion: The remaining 50% is excreted in urine as unchanged drug. The metabolites are excreted through the lungs as carbon dioxide and in urine as urea.

Contraindications and precautions

Hydroxyurea is a toxic drug. Therapeutic response is usually accompanied by toxicity. At daily dosages of 40 mg/kg, about 67% of patients are likely to experience some form of toxicity; all patients experience toxicity at 80 mg/kg. Drug-induced myelosuppression may leave patients susceptible to hemorrhagic complications or viral, bacterial, or fungal infections.

Hydroxyurea is contraindicated in patients with a WBC count below $2,500/mm^3$, in those with a platelet count below $100,000/mm^3$, and in severely anemic patients because of the drug's hematologic toxicity. It is also contraindicated in pregnant patients because it may be fetotoxic.

Hydroxyurea should be used with extreme caution in patients with impaired renal function; they are susceptible to the development of visual and auditory hallucinations and pronounced hematologic toxicity.

Interactions

Concomitant use of fluorouracil with hydroxyurea may decrease the activity of fluorouracil. Hydroxyurea appears to inhibit the conversion of fluorouracil to its active metabolite. A high incidence of neurotoxicity may occur when these two agents are administered together.

Effects on diagnostic tests

Hydroxyurea therapy elevates BUN, serum creatinine, and serum uric acid levels.

---

*Canada only   †Off-label use   Italicized adverse reactions are life-threatening.

Adverse reactions

CNS: drowsiness, hallucinations, *seizures,* headache.
DERM: rash, pruritus, facial erythema.
GI: anorexia, nausea, vomiting, diarrhea, stomatitis, constipation.
GU: increased BUN and serum creatinine levels.
HEMA: *bone marrow depression* (dose-limiting), *leukopenia, thrombocytopenia,* anemia, megaloblastosis.
Metabolic: hyperuricemia.
Other: alopecia.
   Note: Drug should be discontinued if inflammation of the mucous membranes is severe, if WBC count is below 2,500/mm^3, or if platelet count is below 100,000/mm^3.

Overdose and treatment

Clinical manifestations of overdose include myelosuppression, ulceration of buccal and GI mucosa, facial erythema, maculopapular rash, disorientation, hallucinations, and impairment of renal tubular function.
   Treatment is usually supportive and includes transfusion of blood components.

Special considerations

- Dose modification may be required following other chemotherapy or radiation therapy. Hydroxyurea may exacerbate postirradiation erythema.
- Monitor intake and output levels; keep patient hydrated.
- Routinely measure BUN, uric acid, and serum creatinine levels.
- Hydroxyurea can impair fertility. Reversible germ cell toxicity has followed treatment with hydroxyurea.
- Auditory and visual hallucinations and blood toxicity increase when decreased renal function exists.
- Avoid all I.M. injections when platelet count is below 100,000/mm^3.
- Store capsules in tight container at room temperature. Avoid exposure to excessive heat.
- Hydroxyurea is currently under investigation for the treatment of sickle cell anemia. Widespread use of the drug for

this disease is not recommended because of the potential for toxicity.
- Children may be more sensitive to the effects of hydroxyurea, requiring a lower dosage.

Information for the patient
- If patient can't swallow capsule, tell him to empty contents into water and take immediately.
- Emphasize importance of continuing medication despite nausea and vomiting.
- Tell patient to call immediately if vomiting occurs shortly after taking a dose.
- Encourage daily fluid intake of ten to twelve 8-oz (240-ml) glasses to increase urine output and facilitate uric acid excretion.
- Tell patient to report unusual bruising or bleeding.
- Tell patient to avoid exposure to persons with infections.

Geriatric use
Elderly patients may be more sensitive to the effects of hydroxyurea, requiring a lower dosage.

---

methylprednisolone (systemic)
Medrol

methylprednisolone acetate
dep-Medalone, Depoject, Depo-Medrol, Depopred, Depo-Predate, Duralone, Durameth, Medralone, Medrone, M-Prednisol, Rep-Pred

methylprednisolone sodium succinate
A-methaPred, Solu-Medrol

Pregnancy risk category: C

How supplied

Methylprednisolone
Tablets: 2 mg, 4 mg, 8 mg, 16 mg, 24 mg, 32 mg
Methylprednisolone acetate
Injection: 20 mg/ml, 40 mg/ml, 80 mg/ml suspension

Methylprednisolone sodium succinate
Injection: 40 mg/vial, 125 mg/vial, 500 mg/vial, 1,000 mg/vial, 2,000 mg/vial

Indications, route, and dosage

Severe inflammation or immunosuppression
Adults: 4 to 48 mg P.O. daily in a single dose or in divided doses.
Children: 117 mcg/kg to 1.66 mg/kg P.O. daily in three or four divided doses.
Methylprednisolone acetate
Adults: 10 to 80 mg I.M. daily, or 4 to 80 mg into joints and soft tissue p.r.n. q 1 to 5 weeks, or 20 to 60 mg intralesionally.
Children: 117 mcg/kg I.M. q 3 days, or 140 to 835 mcg/kg I.M. q 12 to 24 hours.
Methylprednisolone sodium succinate
Adults: 10 to 250 mg I.M. or I.V. q 4 hours.
Children: 0.03 to 0.2 mg/kg or 1 to 6.25 mg/m^2 I.M. or I.V. daily in divided doses.

Pharmacodynamics

Methylprednisolone stimulates the synthesis of enzymes needed to decrease the inflammatory response. It suppresses the immune system by reducing activity and volume of the lymphatic system, thus producing lymphocytopenia (primarily of T cells); decreasing immunoglobulin and complement concentrations; decreasing passage of immune complexes through basement membranes; and possibly by depressing reactivity of tissue to antigen-antibody interactions.

Methylprednisolone is an intermediate-acting glucocorticoid. It has essentially no mineralocorticoid activity but is a potent glucocorticoid, with five times the potency of an equal weight of hydrocortisone. It is used primarily as an anti-inflammatory agent and immunosuppressant.

Methylprednisolone may be administered orally. Methylprednisolone sodium succinate may be administered by I.M. or I.V. injection or by I.V. infusion, usually at 4- to 6-hour intervals.

Pharmacokinetics

Absorption: Methylprednisolone is absorbed readily after oral administration. After oral and I.V. administration, peak effects occur in about 1 to 2 hours. The acetate suspension for injection has a variable absorption over 24 to 48 hours, depending on whether it is injected into an intra-articular space or a muscle and on the blood supply.

Distribution: Methylprednisolone is distributed rapidly to muscle, liver, skin, intestines, and kidneys. It is distributed into breast milk and through the placenta.

Metabolism: Methylprednisolone is metabolized in the liver to inactive glucuronide and sulfate metabolites.

Excretion: The inactive metabolites and small amounts of unmetabolized drug are excreted by the kidneys. Insignificant quantities of methylprednisolone are excreted in feces. The biological half-life of methylprednisolone is about 18 to 36 hours.

Contraindications and precautions

Methylprednisolone is contraindicated in patients with hypersensitivity to ingredients of adrenocorticoid preparations, and in those with systemic fungal infections (except in adrenal insufficiency). Patients who are receiving methylprednisolone should not be given live virus vaccines because methylprednisolone suppresses the immune response. Glucocorticoids may cause fetal damage if administered to pregnant patients.

Methylprednisolone should be used with extreme caution in patients with GI ulceration, renal disease, hypertension, osteoporosis, diabetes mellitus, thromboembolic disorders, seizures, myasthenia gravis, CHF, tuberculosis, hypoalbuminemia, hypothyroidism, cirrhosis of the liver, emotional instability, psychotic tendencies, hyperlipidemias, glaucoma, or cataracts, because the drug may exacerbate these conditions.

Because adrenocorticoids increase the susceptibility to and mask symptoms of infection, methylprednisolone should not be used (except in life-threatening situations) in patients with viral or bacterial infections not controlled by anti-infective agents.

Interactions

When used concomitantly with anticoagulants, methylprednisolone may decrease the effects of oral anticoagulants by unknown mechanisms.

Methylprednisolone increases the metabolism of isoniazid and salicylates. It causes hyperglycemia, requiring dosage adjustment of insulin or oral antidiabetic drugs in diabetic patients. It may enhance hypokalemia associated with diuretic or amphotericin B therapy. The hypokalemia may increase the risk of toxicity in patients concurrently receiving digitalis glycosides.

Barbiturates, phenytoin, and rifampin may cause decreased corticosteroid effects because of increased hepatic metabolism. Cholestyramine, colestipol, and antacids decrease the corticosteroid effect by adsorbing methylprednisolone, decreasing the amount absorbed.

Concomitant use with estrogens may reduce the metabolism of methylprednisolone by increasing the concentration of transcortin. The half-life of methylprednisolone is then prolonged because of increased protein binding. Concomitant administration of methylprednisolone and ulcerogenic drugs such as NSAIDs may increase the risk of GI ulceration.

Effects on diagnostic tests

Methylprednisolone suppresses reactions to skin tests. It causes false-negative results in the nitroblue tetrazolium test for systemic bacterial infections, and decreases iodine 131 uptake and protein-bound iodine concentrations in thyroid function tests. Methylprednisolone may increase glucose and cholesterol levels; may decrease serum potassium, calcium, thyroxine, and triiodothyronine levels; and may increase urine glucose and calcium levels.

Adverse reactions

When administered in high doses or for prolonged therapy, methylprednisolone suppresses release of corticotropin from the pituitary gland; in turn, the adrenal cortex stops secreting endogenous corticosteroids. The degree and duration of hypothalamic-pituitary-adrenal (HPA) axis suppression produced by methylprednisolone is highly variable among patients and depends on the dose, frequency and time of

---

*Canada only   †Off-label use   Italicized adverse reactions are life-threatening.

administration, and duration of methylprednisolone therapy.

CNS: euphoria, insomnia, headache, psychotic behavior, pseudotumor cerebri, mental changes, nervousness, restlessness.

CV: CHF, hypertension, edema.

DERM: delayed healing, acne, skin eruptions, striae.

EENT: cataracts, glaucoma, thrush.

GI: peptic ulcer, irritation, increased appetite.

Immune: immunosuppression, increased susceptibility to infection.

Metabolic: hypokalemia, sodium retention, fluid retention, weight gain, hyperglycemia, osteoporosis, growth suppression in children.

Musculoskeletal: muscle atrophy, weakness.

Other: pancreatitis, hirsutism, cushingoid symptoms, withdrawal syndrome (nausea, fatigue, anorexia, dyspnea, hypotension, hypoglycemia, myalgia, arthralgia, fever, dizziness, and fainting). Sudden withdrawal may be fatal or may exacerbate the underlying disease. *Acute adrenal insufficiency* may occur with increased stress (infection, surgery, trauma) or abrupt withdrawal after long-term therapy.

Overdose and treatment

Acute ingestion, even in massive doses, is rarely a clinical problem. Toxic signs and symptoms rarely occur if drug is used for less than 3 weeks, even at large doses. However, chronic use causes adverse physiologic effects, including suppression of the HPA axis, cushingoid appearance, muscle weakness, and osteoporosis.

Special considerations

- Certain injectable forms contain sulfites, which can cause an allergic reaction in sensitive patients. If the patient is sensitive to sulfites, be sure to notify the pharmacy.
- Discard reconstituted solutions after 48 hours.
- Give a daily dose in the morning for better results and less toxicity.
- For I.V. injection, use only methylprednisolone sodium succinate; never use the acetate form. Reconstitute accord-

ing to the manufacturer's directions using the supplied diluent or use bacteriostatic water for injection.

- When administering as direct injection, inject diluted drug into a vein or free-flowing compatible I.V. solution over at least 1 minute. In shock, give massive doses over at least 10 minutes to prevent cardiac arrhythmias and circulatory collapse.
- When administering as an intermittent or continuous infusion, dilute solution according to manufacturer's instructions and give over the prescribed duration. If used for continuous infusion, change solution every 24 hours. Compatible solutions include dextrose 5% in water, 0.9% sodium chloride injection, and dextrose 5% in 0.9% sodium chloride injection.
- Give I.M. injection deep into the gluteal muscle. Avoid S.C. injection because atrophy and sterile abscesses may occur.
- If elderly patients have osteoporosis, the condition may be worsened by methylprednisolone therapy. Patients receiving long-term therapy should consider exercise or physical therapy. Vitamin D or calcium supplements may be useful.
- Gradually reduce drug dosage after long-term therapy.
- Dermal atrophy may occur with large doses of the acetate salt. Use multiple small injections rather than a single large dose, and rotate injection sites.
- Monitor weight, blood pressure, serum electrolyte levels, and sleep patterns. Euphoria may initially interfere with sleep.
- Methylprednisolone may mask or exacerbate infections.
- Watch for depression or psychotic episodes, especially in patients receiving high-dose therapy.
- Patients with diabetes may need increased insulin; monitor blood glucose level.
- Unless contraindicated, give low-sodium diet high in potassium and protein. A potassium supplement may be needed. Monitor for additional potassium depletion from diuretics and amphotericin B.
- Give oral doses with food when possible. Critically ill patients may require concomitant antacid or histamine-2 antagonist therapy.
- Patients with hypothyroidism or cirrhosis may show an enhanced response to the drug.

• Methylprednisolone may be used for alternate-day therapy.

Information for the patient
• Teach patient signs of early adrenal insufficiency, such as fatigue, muscular weakness, joint pain, fever, anorexia, nausea, dyspnea, dizziness, and fainting.
• Tell patient not to discontinue drug abruptly or without doctor's consent.
• Tell patient to take daily dose in the morning for better results and less toxicity.
• Warn patients on long-term therapy about cushingoid symptoms.
• Instruct patient to carry a card identifying his need for supplemental systemic glucocorticoids during stress.

paclitaxel
Taxol
Pregnancy risk category: D

How supplied
Injection: 30 mg/5 ml

Indications, route, and dosage
Ovarian cancer
Women: 135 mg/m² by continuous I.V. infusion over 24 hours. Repeat q 3 weeks until response is seen.
Non-small-cell lung cancer
Adults: 200 mg/m² by continuous I.V infusion over 24 hours. Repeat q 3 weeks.

Pharmacodynamics
A derivative of the western yew evergreen tree *Taxus brevifolia,* paclitaxel blocks mitosis in the G₂ and M phase of the cell cycle. Paclitaxel appears to enhance the assembly of cellular microtubules and prevent their depolymerization.

Pharmacokinetics
Absorption: Paclitaxel is administered I.V.

Distribution: Paclitaxel demonstrates extensive extravascular distribution or tissue binding. Plasma levels remain above 85 ng/ml for 6 to 12 days following an infusion.

Metabolism: Paclitaxel is extensively metabolized, probably in the liver.

Excretion: Paclitaxel is excreted through the bile; 1.3% to 12.6% of a dose are found unchanged in the urine. Terminal half-life ranges from 5.3 to 17.4 hours.

Contraindications and precautions

Hematologic toxicity limits dosage. Patients who have received substantial chemotherapy or radiation therapy before treatment with paclitaxel may require lower doses of drug because pretreatment may enhance toxicity.

Interactions

When administered following cisplatin, paclitaxel excretion is decreased about 33%. There is some evidence that ketoconazole may impair the absorption of paclitaxel.

Effects on diagnostic tests

Blood and urine uric acid concentrations may be increased; serum creatinine and BUN levels may be altered.

Adverse reactions

CNS: headache, fatigue, peripheral neuropathy.
CV: bradycardia.
GI: diarrhea, nausea, vomiting, mucositis.
HEMA: *neutropenia,* thrombocytopenia, leukopenia.
Other: alopecia, arthralgia, myalgia, fever, taste perversion, hypersensitivity reactions (dyspnea, bronchospasm, hypotension, urticaria, and erythematous rashes).

Special considerations

All information is based on current literature. Dosage, indications, and adverse effects can change with additional clinical experience.

• Most adverse reactions to paclitaxel are dose related. Neutropenia is significant but transient (less than 10 days in

clinical trials). In one study, all patients developed complete alopecia.
- Hypersensitivity reactions are minimized by infusing the drug over 24 hours and pretreating the patient with antihistamines or corticosteroids. These adverse reactions may be caused by polyoxyethylated castor oil, the vehicle for the drug.
- Paclitaxel is in extremely short supply; 25,000 lb of tree bark yields only 1 kg of drug, and most patients need 1.2 to 1.5 kg for a full course of therapy. Several alternatives are being investigated, including both naturally occurring and synthetic derivatives of the drug, synthetic cultures of the tree, and taxotere, an extract of the needles of the tree.

Information for the patient
Encourage the patient to report adverse reactions, especially easy bruising or bleeding.

prednisone
Apo-Prednisone*, Meticorten, Novoprednisone*, Orasone, Panasol, Prednicen-M, Winpred*
Pregnancy risk category: C

How supplied

Tablets: 1 mg, 2.5 mg, 5 mg, 10 mg, 20 mg, 25 mg, 50 mg
Oral solution: 5 mg/ml, 5 mg/5 ml
Syrup: 5 mg/5 ml

Indications, route, and dosage

Severe inflammation or immunosuppression
Adults: 5 to 60 mg P.O. daily in single dose or divided doses. (Maximum daily dose is 250 mg.) Maintenance dose given once daily or every other day. Dosage must be individualized.
Children: 0.14 mg/kg or 4 to 6 mg/m² P.O. daily in divided doses; alternatively, may use the following dosage schedule:
—*Children age 11 to 18:* 20 mg P.O. q.i.d.
—*Children age 5 to 10:* 15 mg P.O. q.i.d.
—*Children age 18 months to 4 years:* 7.5 to 10 mg P.O. q.i.d.

Pharmacodynamics

Prednisone stimulates the synthesis of enzymes needed to decrease the inflammatory response. It suppresses the immune system by reducing the activity and volume of the lymphatic system, thus producing lymphocytopenia (primarily of T cells); decreasing immunoglobulin and complement concentrations; decreasing passage of immune complexes through basement membranes; and possibly by depressing reactivity of tissue to antigen-antibody interactions.

Prednisone is one of the intermediate-acting glucocorticoids, with greater glucocorticoid activity than cortisone and hydrocortisone, but less anti-inflammatory activity than betamethasone, dexamethasone, and paramethasone. Prednisone is about four to five times more potent as an anti-inflammatory agent than hydrocortisone, but it has only half the mineralocorticoid activity of an equal weight of hydrocortisone. Prednisone is the oral glucocorticoid of choice for anti-inflammatory or immunosuppressant effects.

Pharmacokinetics

Absorption: Prednisone is absorbed readily after oral administration, with peak effects occurring in about 1 to 2 hours.
Distribution: Prednisone is distributed rapidly to muscle, liver, skin, intestines, and kidneys. Prednisone is extensively bound to plasma proteins (transcortin and albumin). Only the unbound portion is active. Prednisone is distributed into breast milk and through the placenta.
Metabolism: Prednisone is metabolized in the liver to the active metabolite prednisolone, which is then metabolized to inactive glucuronide and sulfate metabolites.
Excretion: The inactive metabolites and small amounts of unmetabolized drug are excreted by the kidneys. Insignificant quantities of prednisone are also excreted in feces. The biological half-life of prednisone is 18 to 36 hours.

Contraindications and precautions

Prednisone is contraindicated in patients with systemic fungal infections (except in adrenal insufficiency) and in those with hypersensitivity to ingredients of adrenocorticoid preparations. Patients receiving prednisone should not be given live virus vaccines because prednisone suppresses the immune response.

Prednisone should be used with extreme caution in patients with GI ulceration, renal disease, hypertension, osteoporosis, diabetes mellitus, thromboembolic disorders, seizures, myasthenia gravis, CHF, tuberculosis, hypoalbuminemia, hypothyroidism, cirrhosis of the liver, emotional instability, psychotic tendencies, hyperlipidemias, glaucoma, or cataracts because the drug may exacerbate these conditions.

Because it increases the susceptibility to and mask symptoms of infection, prednisone should not be used (except in life-threatening situations) in patients with viral or bacterial infections not controlled by anti-infective agents.

Interactions

Concomitant use of prednisone with oral anticoagulants rarely may decrease the effects of oral anticoagulants by unknown mechanisms.

Prednisone increases the metabolism of isoniazid and salicylates. It causes hyperglycemia, requiring dosage adjustment of insulin or oral antidiabetic drugs in diabetic patients. Prednisone may enhance the hypokalemia associated with diuretic or amphotericin B therapy. The hypokalemia may increase the risk of toxicity in patients concurrently receiving digitalis glycosides.

Barbiturates, phenytoin, and rifampin may cause decreased prednisone effects because of increased hepatic metabolism. Cholestyramine, colestipol, and antacids decrease the effect of prednisone by adsorbing the corticosteroid, decreasing the amount absorbed.

Concomitant use with estrogens may reduce the metabolism of prednisone by increasing the concentration of transcortin. The half-life of prednisone is then prolonged because of increased protein binding.

Concomitant administration of ulcerogenic drugs such as NSAIDs and prednisone may increase the risk of GI ulceration.

Effects on diagnostic tests

Prednisone suppresses reactions to skin tests. It causes false-negative results in the nitroblue tetrazolium test for systemic bacterial infections, and decreases iodine 131 uptake and protein-bound iodine concentrations in thyroid function tests. Prednisone may increase glucose and cholesterol levels and decrease serum potassium, calcium, thyroxine, and triiodothyronine levels; and may increase urine glucose and calcium levels.

Adverse reactions

When administered in high doses or for prolonged therapy, prednisone suppresses release of ACTH from the pituitary gland. In turn, the adrenal cortex stops secreting endogenous corticosteroids. The degree and duration of hypothalamic-pituitary-adrenal (HPA) axis suppression produced by prednisone is highly variable among patients and depends on the dose, frequency and time of administration, and duration of prednisone therapy.

CNS: euphoria, insomnia, headache, psychotic behavior, pseudotumor cerebri, mental changes, nervousness, restlessness.

CV: *CHF,* hypertension, edema.

DERM: delayed healing, acne, skin eruptions, striae.

EENT: cataracts, glaucoma, thrush.

GI: peptic ulcer, gastric irritation, increased appetite.

Immune: increased susceptibility to infection.

Metabolic: hypokalemia, sodium retention, fluid retention, weight gain, hyperglycemia, osteoporosis, growth suppression in children.

Musculoskeletal: muscle atrophy, weakness.

Other: *pancreatitis,* hirsutism, cushingoid symptoms, withdrawal syndrome (nausea, fatigue, anorexia, dyspnea, hypotension, hypoglycemia, myalgia, arthralgia, fever, dizziness, and fainting). Sudden withdrawal may be fatal or may exacerbate the underlying disease. *Acute adrenal insufficiency* may occur with increased stress (infection, surgery, trauma) or abrupt withdrawal after long-term therapy.

Overdose and treatment

Acute ingestion, even in massive doses, is rarely a clinical problem. Toxic signs and symptoms rarely occur if drug is used for less than 3 weeks, even at large dosages. However, chronic use causes adverse physiologic effects, including suppression of the HPA axis, cushingoid appearance, muscle weakness, and osteoporosis.

Special considerations

- Gradually reduce drug dosage after long-term therapy.
- Monitor weight, blood pressure, serum electrolyte levels, and sleep patterns. Euphoria may initially interfere with sleep.
- Prednisone may mask or exacerbate infections.
- Give daily dosage in the morning for better results and less toxicity.
- Watch for depression or psychotic episodes, especially in patients receiving high-dose therapy.
- Patients with diabetes may need increased insulin; monitor blood glucose levels.
- Unless contraindicated, give low-sodium diet high in potassium and protein. Potassium supplement may also be needed. Watch for additional potassium depletion from diuretics and amphotericin B.
- Give dose with food when possible. Critically ill patients may require concomitant antacid or histamine-2 antagonist therapy.
- For those patients who cannot swallow tablets, liquid forms are available. The oral concentrate (5 mg/ml) may be diluted in juice or another flavored diluent or mixed in semisolid food (such as applesauce) before administration.
- Patients with hypothyroidism or cirrhosis may show an enhanced response to the drug.
- Patients receiving long-term therapy should consider exercise or physical therapy to maintain bone strength. Vitamin D or calcium supplements may also be useful.
- Prednisone may be used for alternate-day therapy.

Information for the patient
- Instruct patient to carry a card identifying his need for supplemental systemic glucocorticoids during stress.

- Stress the importance of taking the drug exactly as prescribed.
- Warn patients on long-term therapy about cushingoid symptoms.
- Tell patient not to discontinue drug abruptly or without doctor's consent.

Geriatric use
Elderly patients may be more susceptible to osteoporosis.

---

teniposide (VM-26)
Vumon*

Pregnancy risk category: D

How supplied

Injection: 50 mg/5 ml ampules

Indications, route, and dosage

Indications and dosage may vary. Check current literature for recommended protocol.
†**Hodgkin's disease and non-Hodgkin's lymphomas, acute lymphocytic leukemia, bladder cancer**
Adults: 50 to 100 mg/m² I.V. once or twice weekly for 4 to 6 weeks, or 40 to 50 mg/m² I.V. daily for 5 days, repeated q 3 to 4 weeks.
Children: 130 mg/m² I.V. weekly, increasing to 150 mg/m² after 3 weeks and to 180 mg/m² after 6 weeks.
†**Neuroblastoma**
Adults: 130 to 180 mg/m² I.V. once weekly.

Pharmacodynamics

Teniposide exerts its cytotoxic activity as a mitotic spindle poison, arresting the cell in metaphase and impairing cellular respiration and energy production.

Pharmacokinetics

Absorption: Teniposide is not administered orally.
Distribution: Teniposide distributes mainly into the liver, kidneys, small intestine, and adrenal glands. The drug is highly

---

*Canada only   †Off-label use   *Italicized adverse reactions are life-threatening.*

bound to plasma proteins. Teniposide crosses the blood-brain barrier to a limited extent.

Metabolism: Teniposide is metabolized extensively in the liver.

Excretion: Approximately 40% of a dose is eliminated through the kidneys as unchanged drug or metabolites. The elimination of teniposide from the plasma is described as triphasic, with half-lives of 45 minutes, 4 hours, and 20 hours for the initial, secondary, and terminal phases, respectively.

Contraindications and precautions

Teniposide is contraindicated in patients with hypersensitivity to podophyllum or semisynthetic podophyllotoxin derivatives.

Interactions

None reported.

Effects on diagnostic tests

Teniposide therapy may increase blood and urine concentrations of uric acid.

Adverse reactions

CV: hypotension from rapid infusion.
GI: nausea and vomiting, diarrhea.
HEMA: *bone marrow depression* (dose-limiting), leukopenia, thrombocytopenia.
Local: chemical thrombophlebitis.
Other: alopecia (rare), *anaphylaxis* (rare), *bronchospasm.*

Overdose and treatment

Clinical manifestations of overdose include myelosuppression, nausea, and vomiting.

   Treatment is usually supportive and includes transfusion of blood components, administration of antiemetics, and administration of antibiotics for any infections that develop.

Special considerations

• Dilute with at least 5 equal volumes (preferably 10 to 20 volumes) of 0.9% sodium chloride solution for I.V. infu-

---

sion. This solution is preferred because of the high incidence of precipitation with dextrose 5% in water.
- Discard cloudy solutions.
- Solutions containing 0.5 to 2 mg/ml are stable for 4 hours. Solutions containing 0.1 to 0.2 mg/ml are stable for 6 hours.
- Teniposide should not be administered through a membrane-type in-line filter because the diluent may dissolve the filter.
- Administer I.V. infusion over at least 45 minutes to prevent hypotension. Avoid I.V. push because of increased risk of hypotension.
- Dosage should be decreased in patients with renal or hepatic insufficiency.
- Monitor for chemical phlebitis at injection site.
- Have diphenhydramine, hydrocortisone, epinephrine, and an airway available in case of an anaphylactic reaction.
- Monitor blood pressure before infusion and at 30-minute intervals during infusion. If systolic blood pressure falls below 90 mm Hg, stop infusion.
- Monitor CBC. Observe patient for signs of bone marrow depression.
- Drug may be given by local bladder instillation to treat bladder cancer.

Information for the patient
- Encourage adequate fluid intake to increase urine output and facilitate uric acid excretion.
- Advise patient to avoid exposure to persons with infections.
- Tell patient that hair should grow back after treatment is discontinued.
- Tell patient to call promptly if he develops a sore throat or fever or notices unusual bruising or bleeding.

---

vinblastine sulfate (VLB)
Velban, Velbe*

Pregnancy risk category: D

How supplied

Injection: 10-mg vials (lyophilized powder), 10 mg/10 ml vials

Indications, route, and dosage

Indications and dosage may vary. Check current literature for recommended protocol.

Breast or testicular cancer, Hodgkin's disease and non-Hodgkin's lymphomas, choriocarcinoma, lymphosarcoma, neuroblastoma, lung cancer, mycosis fungoides, histiocytosis, Kaposi's sarcoma

Adults: 0.1 mg/kg or 3.7 mg/m² I.V. weekly or q 2 weeks. May be increased in weekly increments of 50 mcg/kg or 1.8 to 1.9 mg/m² to maximum dose of 0.5 mg/kg or 18.5 mg/m² I.V. weekly, according to response. Dose should not be repeated if WBC count falls below 4,000/mm³.

Children: 2.5 mg/m² I.V. as a single dose every week, increased weekly in increments of 1.25 mg/m² to a maximum of 7.5 mg/m².

Pharmacodynamics

Vinblastine exerts its cytotoxic activity by arresting the cell cycle in the metaphase portion of cell division, resulting in a blockade of mitosis. The drug also inhibits DNA-dependent RNA synthesis and interferes with amino acid metabolism, inhibiting purine synthesis.

Pharmacokinetics

Absorption: Vinblastine is absorbed unpredictably across the GI tract after oral administration, which is why it must be given I.V.

Distribution: Vinblastine is distributed widely into body tissues. The drug crosses the blood-brain barrier but does not achieve therapeutic concentrations in the CSF.

Metabolism: Vinblastine is metabolized partially in the liver to an active metabolite.

---

*Canada only   †Off-label use   Italicized adverse reactions are life-threatening.

Excretion: Vinblastine is excreted primarily in bile as unchanged drug. A smaller portion is excreted in urine. The plasma elimination of vinblastine is described as triphasic, with half-lives of 35 minutes, 53 minutes, and 19 hours for the alpha, beta, and terminal phases, respectively.

Contraindications and precautions

Vinblastine is contraindicated in patients with severe leukopenia or bacterial infections because treatment with myelosuppressive drugs such as vinblastine causes an increased frequency of infections.

Interactions

Concomitant use of vinblastine with methotrexate increases the effect of methotrexate by increasing cellular uptake of methotrexate. This interaction allows a lower dose of methotrexate, reducing the potential for methotrexate toxicity.

Effects on diagnostic tests

Vinblastine therapy may increase blood and urine concentrations of uric acid.

Adverse reactions

CNS: depression, paresthesias, peripheral neuropathy and neuritis, numbness, loss of deep tendon reflexes, muscle pain and weakness.
DERM: dermatitis, vesiculation.
EENT: pharyngitis.
GI: nausea, vomiting, stomatitis, ulcer, GI bleeding, constipation, ileus, anorexia, weight loss, abdominal pain. *(Note:* Drug should be discontinued if patient develops stomatitis.)
GU: oligospermia, aspermia, urine retention.
HEMA: *bone marrow depression* (dose-limiting), *leukopenia* (nadir on days 4 to 10 and lasts another 7 to 14 days), *thrombocytopenia.*
Local: irritation, phlebitis, cellulitis, necrosis if I.V. extravasates.
Other: *acute bronchospasm,* reversible alopecia (in 5% to 10% of patients), pain in tumor site, low fever.

---

*Canada only   †Off-label use   Italicized adverse reactions are life-threatening.

Overdose and treatment

Clinical manifestations of overdose include stomatitis, ileus, mental depression, paresthesias, loss of deep tendon reflexes, permanent CNS damage, and myelosuppression.

Treatment is usually supportive and includes transfusion of blood components and appropriate symptomatic therapy.

Special considerations

Besides those relevant to all vinca alkaloids, consider the following recommendations.

- To reconstitute drug, use 10 ml of preserved 0.9% sodium chloride injection to yield a concentration of 1 mg/ml.
- Vinblastine may be administered by I.V. push injection over 1 minute into the tubing of a free-flowing I.V. infusion.
- Dilution into larger volume is not recommended for infusion into peripheral veins. This method increases risk of extravasation. Vinblastine may be administered as an I.V. infusion through a central venous catheter.
- To reduce nausea, give an antiemetic before administering vinblastine.
- Do not administer more frequently than every 7 days to allow review of effect on WBCs before administration of next dose. Leukopenia may develop.
- Reduced dosage may be required in patients with liver disease.
- After administering, monitor for life-threatening acute bronchospasm reaction. This reaction is most likely to occur in a patient who is also receiving mitomycin.
- Prevent uric acid nephropathy with generous oral fluid intake and administration of allopurinol.
- Monitor WBC, RBC, and platelet counts, and hemoglobin level weekly during therapy.
- Treat extravasation with liberal injection of hyaluronidase into the site, followed by warm compresses to minimize the spread of the reaction. (Some clinicians treat extravasation with cold compresses.) Prepare hyaluronidase by adding 3 ml of 0.9% sodium chloride solution to the 150-unit vial.
- Give laxatives as needed. Stool softeners may be used prophylactically.

- Do not confuse vinblastine with vincristine or the investigational agent vindesine.
- Vinblastine is less neurotoxic than vincristine.

Information for the patient
- Encourage adequate fluid intake to increase urine output and facilitate uric acid excretion.
- Reassure patient that therapeutic response is not immediate. Adequate trial is 12 weeks.
- Advise patient to avoid exposure to persons with infections.
- Reassure patient that hair should grow back after treatment has ended.
- Instruct patients to report any symptoms of sore throat and fever and of unusual bruising or bleeding.

Geriatric use
Patients with cachexia or ulceration of the skin (which is more common in elderly patients) may be more susceptible to the leukopenic effect of this drug.

vincristine sulfate
Oncovin
Pregnancy risk category: D

How supplied
Injection: 1 mg/ml, 2 mg/2 ml, 5 mg/5 ml multiple-dose vials; 1 mg/ml, 2 mg/2 ml preservative-free vials

Indications, route, and dosage
Indications and dosage may vary. Check current literature for recommended protocol.
Acute lymphoblastic and other leukemias; Hodgkin's disease; lymphosarcoma; reticulum cell, osteogenic, and other sarcomas; neuroblastoma; rhabdomyosarcoma; Wilms' tumor; lung and breast cancers
Adults: 10 to 30 mcg/kg or 0.4 to 1.4 mg/m² I.V. weekly.
Children: 1.5 to 2 mg/m² I.V. weekly. Maximum single dose (adults and children) is 2 mg.
—Children under 10 kg or <1 m²: 0.05 mg/kg I.V. once weekly.

Pharmacodynamics

Vincristine exerts its cytotoxic activity by arresting the cell cycle in the metaphase portion of cell division, resulting in a blockade of mitosis. The drug also inhibits DNA-dependent RNA synthesis and interferes with amino acid metabolites, inhibiting purine synthesis.

Pharmacokinetics

Absorption: Vincristine is absorbed unpredictably across the GI tract after oral administration and therefore must be given I.V.

Distribution: Vincristine is rapidly and widely distributed into body tissues and is bound to RBCs and platelets. The drug crosses the blood-brain barrier but does not achieve therapeutic concentrations in the CSF.

Metabolism: Vincristine is extensively metabolized in the liver.

Excretion: Vincristine and its metabolites are primarily excreted into bile. A smaller portion is eliminated through the kidneys. The plasma elimination of vincristine is described as triphasic, with half-lives of about 4 minutes, $2^1/_4$ hours, and 85 hours for the distribution, second, and terminal phases, respectively.

Contraindications and precautions

Vincristine is contraindicated in patients with the demyelinating form of Charcot-Marie-Tooth syndrome because of the drug's neurotoxic effects. Vincristine is also contraindicated in patients with hepatic failure and in those receiving radiation therapy through ports that include the liver.

Use with caution in patients with preexisting neuromuscular disease, closely monitoring for neurotoxicity. Also use cautiously in patients receiving other neurotoxic drugs. Use cautiously in patients with jaundice or hepatic dysfunction.

Interactions

Concomitant use of vincristine with methotrexate increases the therapeutic effect of methotrexate. This interaction may be used to therapeutic advantage; it allows a lower dose of methotrexate, reducing the potential for methotrexate toxicity. Concomitant use with other neurotoxic drugs increases neurotoxicity through an additive effect.

Asparaginase decreases the hepatic clearance of vincristine. Calcium channel blockers enhance vincristine accumulation in cells. Concomitant use of vincristine with digoxin decreases digoxin levels; monitor serum digoxin levels. Use with mitomycin may possibly increase the frequency of bronchospasm and acute pulmonary reactions.

Effects on diagnostic tests

Vincristine therapy may increase blood and urine concentrations of uric acid and serum potassium.

Adverse reactions

CNS: neurotoxicity (dose-limiting), peripheral neuropathy, sensory loss, deep tendon reflex loss, paresthesias, wristdrop and footdrop, ataxia, cranial nerve palsies (headache, jaw pain, hoarseness, vocal cord paralysis, visual disturbances), muscle weakness and cramps, depression, agitation, insomnia; some neurotoxicities may be permanent.
EENT: diplopia, optic and extraocular neuropathy, ptosis.
GI: constipation, cramps, ileus that mimics surgical abdomen, nausea, vomiting, anorexia, stomatitis, weight loss, dysphagia, *intestinal necrosis*.
GU: urine retention.
HEMA: rapidly reversible mild anemia and *leukopenia*.
Local: severe local reaction when extravasated, phlebitis, cellulitis.
Other: *acute bronchospasm*, reversible alopecia (in up to 71% of patients), SIADH.

Overdose and treatment

Clinical manifestations of overdose include alopecia, myelosuppression, paresthesias, neuritic pain, motor difficulties, loss of deep tendon reflexes, nausea, vomiting, and ileus.

Treatment is usually supportive and includes transfusion of blood components; administration of antiemetics, enemas for ileus, or phenobarbital for seizures; and other appropriate symptomatic therapy. Administration of leucovorin calcium at a dosage of 15 mg I.V. every 3 hours for 24 hours,

---

then every 6 hours for 48 hours, may help protect cells from the toxic effects of vincristine.

Special considerations

Besides those relevant to all vinca alkaloids, consider the following recommendations.

- Vincristine may be administered by I.V. push injection over 1 minute into the tubing of a free-flowing I.V. infusion.
- Dilution into larger volumes is not recommended for infusion into peripheral veins; this increases risk of extravasation. Vincristine may be administered as an I.V. infusion through a central venous catheter.
- Necrosis may result from extravasation. Manufacturer recommends treatment with cold compresses and prompt administration of 150 units of intradermal hyaluronidase, sodium bicarbonate, and local injection of hydrocortisone, or a combination of these treatments. However, some clinicians prefer to treat extravasation with warm compresses only.
- After administering, monitor for life-threatening bronchospasm reaction. It is most likely to occur in a patient who is also receiving mitomycin.
- Because of potential for neurotoxicity, do not give vincristine more than once a week. Children are more resistant to neurotoxicity than adults. Neurotoxicity is dose-related and usually reversible; reduce dose if symptoms of neurotoxicity develop.
- Check WBC and hemoglobin level before each dose.
- Monitor for neurotoxicity by checking for depression of Achilles tendon reflex, numbness, tingling, footdrop or wrist-drop, difficulty in walking, ataxia, and slapping gait. Also check ability to walk on heels. Patient should have support while walking.
- Prevent uric acid nephropathy with generous oral fluid intake and administration of allopurinol. Alkalinization of urine may be required if serum uric acid concentration is increased.
- Monitor bowel function. Give patient stool softener, laxative, or water before dosing. Constipation may be an early sign of neurotoxicity.

- Patients with obstructive jaundice or liver disease should receive a reduced dosage.
- Be sure to avoid confusing vincristine with vinblastine or the investigational agent vindesine.
- Vials of 5 mg are for multiple-dose use only. Do not administer entire vial to patient as single dose.
- Drug may cause SIADH. Treatment requires fluid restriction and a loop diuretic.

Information for the patient

- Encourage adequate fluid intake to increase urine output and facilitate uric acid excretion.
- Tell patient to call regarding use of laxatives if constipation or stomach pain occurs.
- Assure patient that hair growth should resume after treatment is discontinued.
- Advise patient to avoid exposure to persons with infections.
- Tell the patient to contact the doctor if sore throat or fever develops.

Geriatric use

Elderly patients who are weak or bedridden may be more susceptible to neurotoxic effects.

Investigational drugs

aclarubicin hydrochloride	piroxantrone hydrochloride
amifostine	prednimustine
amsacrine	sodium suramin
buserelin acetate	sparfosate sodium
dexrazoxane	taxotere
edatrexate	topotecan
epirubicin hydrochloride	toremifene citrate
irinotecan	vindesine sulfate
menogaril	vinorelbine ditartrate
mitoguazone	

The following drugs may be available through investigational protocols. The information presented here is limited to currently available information. Please note that published data are not consistently available regarding drug interactions, known interference with laboratory tests, and contraindications and precautions. Contact the product manufacturer for more information.

aclarubicin hydrochloride (aclacinomycin A hydrochloride, NSC-208734)
Aclacin

How supplied

Available only through investigational protocols

Indications, route, and dosage

Acute nonlymphocytic leukemia
Adults: 175 to 300 mg/m² I.V. in divided doses over 3 to 7 days. Alternatively, may be given as a single infusion of 25 to 100 mg/m² I.V. q 3 to 4 weeks. Cumulative dose is usually 300 to 600 mg/m².

Dosages may be reduced when given as part of combination therapy.

Pharmacodynamics

Aclarubicin is an anthracycline antibiotic that exerts its cytotoxic activity by intercalating between DNA base pairs and uncoiling the DNA helix. The result is inhibition of DNA synthesis and DNA-dependent RNA synthesis.

Adverse reactions

CV: ECG changes, *cardiotoxicity, cardiomyopathy* (rare).
DERM: alopecia.
GI: nausea, vomiting, mucositis.
HEMA: *bone-marrow depression* (dose-limiting), thrombocytopenia, neutropenia, leukopenia.

Special considerations

- Mix injections with 0.9% sodium chloride injection.
- Bone marrow depression may be more pronounced in patients who have received mitomycin or a nitrosourea.
- Aclarabucin probably has less cardiotoxicity and causes less alopecia than doxorubicin, but GI toxicity and mucositis are at least as common and may be more severe.

amifostine (ethiofos, WR-2721)
Ethyol

How supplied

Available under investigational protocols from the National Cancer Institute or U.S. Bioscience
Injection: 500 mg/vial

Indications, route, and dosage

Reduction of toxicity caused by radiation or alkylating agents such as cisplatin
Adults: 740 to 910 mg/m^2 I.V. 15 to 30 minutes before treatment with alkylating agent or radiation.

Pharmacodynamics

Amifostine preferentially distributes into normal tissues such as GI mucosa, skin, and bone marrow but not into tumor tissue. The drug provides free sulfhydryl groups that scavenge potentially toxic metabolites formed from radiation therapy or chemotherapy.

Pharmacokinetics

Absorption: Amifostine is undetectable in plasma within 6 minutes of injection.
Distribution: Amifostine is preferentially distributed to normal tissue rather than tumor tissue.
Metabolism: Amifostine is nearly completely metabolized.
Excretion: Less than 3% of amifostine is found in the urine unchanged.

Contraindications and precautions

Because amifostine may cause hypotension, use cautiously with drugs that may exacerbate hypotension, such as benzodiazepines.

Adverse reactions

CNS: somnolence.
CV: transient hypotension, flushing.
GI: nausea, *vomiting* (may be severe).
Other: hypocalcemia.

Special considerations

- Premedicate patient with an antiemetic because nausea and vomiting may be severe.
- Store unopened vials in the refrigerator or freezer. Reconstituted drug is stable at room temperature for 8 hours.
- Reconstitute vial with 9.3 ml sterile water for injection to yield a solution of 50 mg/ml. Further dilute to 10 mg/ml

---

*Canada only   †Off-label use   Italicized adverse reactions are life-threatening.

with dextrose 5% in water or 0.9% sodium chloride injection. Diluted drug is stable for 24 hours at room temperature.
- Amifostine has been investigated in the management of hypercalcemia, but adverse effects and lack of efficacy have limited its use.

amsacrine (m-AMSA)
Amsa P-D*

Pregnancy risk category: C

How supplied

Available under investigational protocols from the National Cancer Institute and Warner-Lambert Company
Injection: 50 mg/ml

Indications, route, and dosage

Indications and dosage may vary. Check current literature for recommended protocol.
Acute adult leukemias
Adults: Induction, 75, 100, or 125 mg/m² I.V. daily infusion (over 60 to 90 minutes) for 5 days. Repeat q 3 to 4 weeks. Maintenance dose, one-half the induction dose, repeated q 7 to 8 weeks.

Pharmacodynamics

Amsacrine exerts its cytotoxic activity by intercalating between DNA base pairs, thus inhibiting DNA synthesis.

Pharmacokinetics

Absorption: Amsacrine is administered I.V. only and is immediately absorbed.
Distribution: Amsacrine is distributed mainly in the liver. It probably does not cross the blood-brain barrier to a significant extent.
Metabolism: Amsacrine is metabolized extensively in the liver.
Excretion: The elimination of amsacrine from the plasma appears to be biphasic, with a half-life of 12 minutes in the ini-

tial phase and $2^{1}/_{2}$ hours in the terminal phase. Amsacrine metabolites are excreted in urine and bile.

Contraindications and precautions

There are no reported contraindications for amsacrine. It should be used cautiously in patients with impaired liver function.

Interactions

Amsacrine and heparin are physically incompatible. Admixture of these two agents results in precipitation.

Effects on diagnostic tests

Amsacrine therapy may increase serum concentrations of bilirubin and alkaline phosphatase, indicating drug-induced cholestasis or hepatotoxicity.

Adverse reactions

CNS: *seizures* at doses as low as 40 mg/m²/day.
CV: *ventricular arrhythmias* and *cardiac arrest* (rare), possibly caused by the diluent.
GI: mild nausea and vomiting, stomatitis at higher doses.
HEMA: *leukopenia* (usually dose-limiting); mild thrombocytopenia; *bone marrow depression* (dose-limiting).
Local: vein irritation, phlebitis.

Overdose and treatment

Clinical manifestations of overdose include myelosuppression, nausea, and vomiting.

Treatment is usually supportive and includes transfusion of blood components and administration of antiemetics.

Special considerations

- To prepare solution for administration, two sterile liquids are combined. Add 1.5 ml from the amsacrine ampule (50 mg/ml) to the vial containing 13.5 ml of lactic acid. The combined solution will contain 5 mg/ml of amsacrine.
- Use a glass syringe for preparation of amsacrine because the alcohol diluent quickly melts plastic unless a buffer is added.

---

*Canada only   †Off-label use   Italicized adverse reactions are life-threatening.

- Solutions for infusion are stable for at least 48 hours at room temperature. Use undiluted mixture within 8 hours; it does not contain a preservative.
- The solution may be further diluted for infusion with dextrose 5% in water (D_5W) to minimize vein irritation. Administer doses of less than 100 mg in at least 100 ml of D_5W; from 100 to 199 mg, in 250 ml D_5W; and of 200 mg or greater, in a minimum of 500 ml D_5W.
- Solutions should be infused slowly over several hours to minimize vein irritation.
- Do not add amsacrine to 0.9% sodium chloride solution or other chloride-containing solutions. Precipitation may occur.
- Do not administer amsacrine through membrane-type in-line filters. The diluent may dissolve the filter.
- Monitor CBC and liver function tests.
- Patient's urine will appear orange.
- Monitor patient closely for CNS and cardiac toxicity during administration.
- Avoid direct contact of amsacrine with skin because of possible sensitization.

Information for the patient
- Encourage adequate fluid intake to increase urine output and to facilitate uric acid excretion.
- Tell patient to avoid exposure to persons with infections.
- Warn patient that amsacrine will turn urine orange.

buserelin acetate (HOE 766)
Suprefact

How supplied

Available only through investigational protocols
Injection: 1 mg/ml
Nasal spray: 10-ml containers

Indications, route, and dosage

Prostate cancer

Men: 500 mcg S.C. t.i.d. for 1 week, then 200 mcg/day S.C. Alternatively, give 800 mcg by intranasal instillation t.i.d. for 1 week, then 400 mcg t.i.d.

Pharmacodynamics

Buserelin, a luteinizing hormone-releasing hormone (LHRH) analog, inhibits gonadotropin release and results in decreased serum concentrations of testosterone. After 1 to 2 weeks, secretion of luteinizing hormone and follicle-stimulating hormone is reduced and serum levels of testosterone approach those seen following castration.

Adverse reactions

CV: hypertension.
DERM: local irritation at injection site, rash.
Endocrine: decreased libido, impotence, gynecomastia in males; cessation of menses and spotting in females.
GI: nausea, vomiting, diarrhea, constipation.
GU: urine retention.
Other: headache; hot flashes; tumor flare at initiation of therapy, possibly resulting in spinal cord compression.

Special considerations

Tumor flare resulting in increased bone pain, urine retention, or spinal cord compression may occur in the first 2 weeks of treatment. Analgesics or antiandrogens, such as flutamide, may be useful.

dexrazoxane (ADR-529)
Zinecard

How supplied

Available under investigational protocols from Adria Laboratories
Injection: 500 mg/vial (lyophilized powder)

Indications, route, and dosage

Prevention of doxorubicin-induced cardiotoxicity
Adults: Dosage is based on the doxorubicin dose and is usually given in a 10:1 to 20:1 ratio. For example, when the doxorubicin dose is 50 mg/m^2, the dexrazoxane dose is 500 to 1,000 mg/m^2 I.V. over 15 to 30 minutes.

Pharmacodynamics

Dexrazoxane, the (+/-) enantiomorph of razoxane, chelates intracellular iron, thus preventing doxorubicin from forming free radicals that promote tissue damage.

Pharmacokinetics

Distribution: Dexrazoxane is widely distributed, and is less than 3% bound to plasma proteins.
Metabolism: Dexrazoxane undergoes hepatic metabolism.
Excretion: 35% to 50% of the drug is excreted in the urine unchanged. Elimination half-life is 2 to 3 hours.

Interactions

When administered concomitantly with doxorubicin, dexrazoxane enhances leukopenia.

Adverse reactions

CNS: fatigue, *seizures.*
CV: hypotension, *deep vein thrombosis.*
GI: nausea, vomiting, anorexia, stomatitis.
HEMA: leukopenia, thrombocytopenia, anemia.
Metabolic: elevated hepatic enzyme levels, hyperbilirubinemia, elevated serum amylase levels, elevated serum triglyceride levels.
Respiratory: *respiratory arrest.*
Other: fever, alopecia.

Special considerations

• In most studies, the incidence and severity of toxicity in patients treated with dexrazoxane plus doxorubicin was similar to that in those treated with doxorubicin alone. Dexrazoxane may slightly enhance leukopenia.

---

*Canada only   †Off-label use   Italicized adverse reactions are life-threatening.

- Dexrazoxane is compatible with solutions containing either dextrose or sodium chloride, or dextrose-sodium chloride combinations. Reconstitute with $^1/_6$ M sodium lactate injection. After reconstitution, drug is stable for 6 hours at room temperature. Dilute in 50 to 100 ml dextrose 5% in water and infuse over 15 to 30 minutes.

edatrexate (10-EDAM, NSC-626715)

How supplied

Available under investigational protocols from the National Cancer Institute
Injection: 50 mg/vial (lyophilized powder)

Indications, route, and dosage

Non-small-cell lung carcinoma, cancers of the head and neck, and other cancers
Adults: 80 mg/m² I.V. bolus weekly.

Pharmacodynamics

Edatrexate is a methotrexate analog that inhibits dihydrofolate reductase.

Pharmacokinetics

Metabolism: Edatrexate is metabolized in the liver to 7-hydroxyedatrexate, which inhibits dihydrofolate reductase.
Excretion: About 33% of a dose appears in the urine. Drug is partially eliminated by renal tubular secretion. Elimination half-life is about 12 hours.

Adverse reactions

CNS: fatigue.
DERM: rash, alopecia (mild).
GI: stomatitis (may be dose-limiting), diarrhea, nausea, vomiting.
HEMA: leukopenia, thrombocytopenia, prolongation of partial thromboplastin and prothrombin times.
Metabolic: elevated hepatic enzyme levels, elevated serum creatinine level.

Respiratory: *interstitial pneumonitis.*

Special considerations

- Edatrexate is classified as an antimetabolite.
- Leucovorin antagonizes the effects of edatrexate. Some studies suggest that leucovorin may limit the stomatitis that edatrexate produces.
- Store vials at room temperature.
- Reconstitute with 4 ml of 0.9% sodium chloride injection. Solution will have a final concentration of 12.5 mg/ml. Administer drug as an I.V. bolus injection over 1 to 2 minutes.

epirubicin hydrochloride (NSC-256942)
Farmorubicin

How supplied

Available under investigational protocols from Adria Laboratories
Injection: 10-mg vials, 50-mg vials

Indications, route, and dosage

Acute leukemias, lymphomas, multiple myeloma, and solid tumors (such as breast, GI tract, or ovarian cancers)

Adults: When used as the sole agent, dosage is 75 to 90 mg/m^2 I.V. q 3 weeks. The dosage may be divided over 2 days. Alternatively, give 20 mg I.V. once weekly. Maximum lifetime cumulative dose is 900 to 1,000 mg/m^2.

Dosage adjustments for patients with hepatic failure: If serum bilirubin level is 12 to 30 mcg/ml, decrease dosage by 50%. If serum bilirubin level is >30 mcg/ml, decrease dosage by 75%.

Pharmacodynamics

Epirubicin is an anthracycline antineoplastic antibiotic with actions similar to those of doxorubicin. It exerts its cytotoxic activity by intercalating between DNA base pairs and uncoiling the DNA helix. The result is inhibition of DNA synthesis and DNA-dependent RNA synthesis.

Pharmacokinetics

Distribution: Following I.V. administration, epirubicin is widely and rapidly distributed throughout tissues. It does not cross the blood-brain barrier.

Metabolism: Epirubicin is metabolized in the liver and excreted mainly in bile; only about 10% of a dose is found in the urine within 48 hours.

Excretion: Plasma elimination half-life is about 40 hours.

Interactions

Epirubicin is incompatible with heparin.

Adverse reactions

CNS: paresthesias, headache, fatigue.
CV: arrhythmias, ECG changes (rarely significant), *CHF.*
DERM: hyperpigmentation of nail beds or dermal creases, dermatitis.
GI: nausea, vomiting, diarrhea, mucositis, anorexia.
HEMA: *leukopenia,* thrombocytopenia, anemia.
Other: *anaphylactoid reactions,* fever, alopecia, red discoloration of urine.

Special considerations

- Decrease dosage in elderly patients and patients who have received previous chemotherapy. Because the drug can promote "radiation recall" skin reactions, use cautiously in patients who have received prior radiation therapy.
- Frequently check blood counts during therapy. Leukopenia is dose-limiting.
- Closely monitor cardiac function.
- Warn the patient that the drug frequently discolors the urine red to reddish brown.

irinotecan (camptothecin-11, CPT-11)

How supplied

Available under investigational protocols from Daiichi Pharmaceutical Company

---

Injection: 20 mg/ml in 2-ml vials, 5-ml vials

Indications, route, and dosage

Carcinoma of the lung (non-small-cell and small-cell); cervix, colon, and ovarian cancers

Adults: Several regimens have been tested, including 100 mg/m^2 I.V. weekly for 3 weeks. Repeat cycle q 4 weeks. Or 125 mg/m^2 I.V. weekly for 4 weeks followed by a 2-week rest period.

Other regimens include 150 mg/m^2 I.V. every other week; 200 to 240 mg/m^2 q 3 to 4 weeks; 40 mg/m^2 for 5 days q 4 weeks; 20 mg/m^2 b.i.d. for 7 days q 4 weeks; 40 mg/m^2 for 3 days every week; or 30 mg/m^2 by continuous I.V. infusion for 5 days q 4 weeks.

When combined with cisplatin (80 mg/m^2 I.V. on day 1 q 4 weeks), dosage is 60 mg/m^2 I.V. weekly (days 1, 8, and 15) for 3 weeks.

Pharmacodynamics

Irinotecan inhibits topoisomerase I, an enzyme that catalyzes the relaxation of supercoiled DNA, an early step in DNA replication.

Pharmacokinetics

Metabolism: Irinotecan is metabolized to 7-ethyl-10-hydroxy-camptothecin (SN-38), an active metabolite that is 40 to 200 times as potent as the parent drug.
Excretion: Elimination of irinotecan is triphasic; elimination half-life is 16 to 18 hours. The metabolite SN-38 has an elimination half-life of 7 to 14 hours.

Contraindications and precautions

Neutropenia is dose limiting and may be severe. The nadir occurs around day 30.

Diarrhea is occasionally severe and unpredictable. Diarrhea usually begins after the second or third dose. Nausea and vomiting occur in 20% to 25% of the patients.

Adverse reactions

CV: bradycardia.

DERM: alopecia, rash.
GI: diarrhea, nausea, vomiting, mucositis, constipation.
GU: elevated serum creatinine levels (rare).
HEMA: *neutropenia* (dose-limiting), eosinophilia, anemia, thrombocytopenia (rare).
Hepatic: elevated AST (formerly SGOT) concentration.
Respiratory: dyspnea, pulmonary infiltrates.
Other: excessive salivation, lacrimation (common); fever, diaphoresis.

Special considerations

- Flushing, cramping, and diarrhea can be significantly reduced by premedication with ondansetron or diphenhydramine with or without atropine.
- The onset of respiratory adverse reactions is delayed and can occur 60 days after beginning treatment.
- Irinotecan is given by I.V. infusion in 500 ml of dextrose 5% in water (D_5W) or 0.9% sodium chloride solution over 90 minutes or longer. When mixed in 500 ml D_5W, solutions are stable at room temperature for at least 24 hours. Solutions shouldn't be refrigerated because drug may precipitate.
- Store at room temperature.

menogaril (7-OMEN, NSC-269148)

How supplied

Available under investigational protocols from the National Cancer Institute and Upjohn
Injection: 50 mg/vial (lyophilized powder)

Indications, route, and dosage

Malignant melanoma, other cancers
Adults: 140 to 200 mg/m^2 I.V. q 3 to 4 weeks; alternatively, administer 50 mg/m^2 daily for 5 days, repeated q 3 to 4 weeks.

Pharmacodynamics

Menogaril is an anthracycline antineoplastic antibiotic derivative with actions similar to those of doxorubicin.

*Canada only   †Off-label use   Italicized adverse reactions are life-threatening.

Pharmacokinetics

Metabolism: Oral bioavailability is limited to 30% because of first-pass hepatic metabolism.

Excretion: Elimination is biphasic or triphasic, with an elimination half-life of about 30 hours. At least one active metabolite, *N*-desmethylmenogaril, has been identified; it has an elimination half-life of about 58 hours. Only 5% of the drug is eliminated in the urine and feces.

Interactions

Menogaril is incompatible with chloride-containing solutions, heparin, and sodium bicarbonate.

Adverse reactions

CNS: malaise.
CV: *CHF*, decreased left ventricular ejection fraction, atrial fibrillation, sinus bradycardia, ventricular extrasystoles.
DERM: alopecia (mild), urticaria, blistering.
GI: nausea, vomiting, diarrhea, mucositis, anorexia.
GU: impotence.
HEMA: *neutropenia,* thrombocytopenia, anemia.
Metabolic: mild elevation of hepatic enzyme levels.
Local: phlebitis, pruritus, inflammation, and pain at the injection site.

Special considerations

- Severity of urticaria is dose-related and may be mild to severe. May be accompanied by blister formation. Neither premedicating with steroids or antihistamines, diluting the drug, nor slowing the infusion rate have had any effect on this adverse reaction.
- Store vials in the refrigerator; protect from light.
- Do not use chloride-containing solutions to reconstitute or dilute drug because of incompatibility. Reconstitute 50-mg vial with 10 ml sterile water to form a solution of 5 mg/ml. Shake well for 2 minutes. Reconstituted solutions are stable for 6 weeks in the refrigerator. Dilute desired dose to a final concentration of 0.1 mg/ml, using dextrose 5% in water.

mitoguazone
[methylglyoxal-bis(guanylhydrazone),
methyl-GAG, NSC-32946]

How supplied

Available under investigational protocols from the National
Cancer Institute
Injection: 1 g/vial (lyophilized powder)

Indications, route, and dosage

**Hodgkin's disease and non-Hodgkin's lymphoma; cutaneous T-cell
lymphoma; multiple myeloma; cancers of the head, neck, esophagus,
and prostate gland**
Adults: 500 mg/m^2 once a week, increasing to 700 mg/m^2
once a week as tolerated.

Pharmacodynamics

Mitoguazone inhibits 5′-adenosylmethionine decarboxylase,
an enzyme important in the synthesis of DNA and RNA.

Pharmacokinetics

Distribution: Mitoguazone rapidly distributes to body water
after I.V. administration, with CSF levels approximately 20%
of plasma levels.
Excretion: Elimination of mitoguazone is triphasic, with the
terminal elimination half-life in excess of 40 hours. Mitoguazone is detectable in plasma 2 weeks after administration. Approximately 15% of the drug is eliminated in the
urine unchanged within 3 days of administration.

Adverse reactions

CNS: malaise, muscle weakness, polyneuropathy, myopathy.
GI: *ileus,* nausea, vomiting, mucositis, diarrhea.
HEMA: leukopenia, thrombocytopenia.
Local: cellulitis, phlebitis after extravasation; vasculitis.
Other: hypoglycemia, facial flushing (during infusion).

Special considerations

- Hypoglycemia is common. Some clinicians advocate administering drug in dextrose 5% in water (D_5W).
- Extravasation may cause severe cellulitis or phlebitis. Be sure to check patency of vein before injection.
- Flushing, especially in the face, is common and may be associated with numbness. Decreasing the infusion rate may lessen the extent and severity of flushing.
- Mucositis is dose limiting and can be severe. May occur in up to 25% of patients receiving weekly treatment.
- Add 9.3 ml 0.9% sodium chloride injection to the 1-g vial to yield a solution of 100 mg/ml. Further dilute in 500 ml D_5W before infusion. Also compatible with 0.9% sodium chloride injection. Infuse over at least 45 minutes.
- Store vials at room temperature. Reconstituted solutions are stable for 48 hours at room temperature. When further diluted, solutions are stable for 7 days.

piroxantrone hydrochloride (oxantrazole hydrochloride, NSC-349174)

How supplied

Available under investigational protocols from the National Cancer Institute
Injection: 50 mg/vial (lyophilized powder)

Indications, route, and dosage

Various cancers
Adults: 150 mg/m² I.V. Repeat q 3 weeks as tolerated.

Pharmacodynamics

Piroxantrone is a structural analog of the anthracycline derivatives. It intercalates between base pairs of DNA and inhibits DNA and RNA synthesis. It also inhibits the actions of topoisomerase II.

Pharmacokinetics

Excretion: Elimination half-life of piroxantrone is about 30 minutes.

Adverse reactions

CNS: fatigue.
CV: *CHF*, heart block, ventricular tachycardia, decreased left ventricular ejection fraction.
DERM: alopecia (infrequent).
GI: anorexia, constipation, diarrhea, nausea, vomiting, mucositis.
HEMA: *leukopenia, thrombocytopenia*.
Metabolic: hyponatremia, elevated hepatic enzyme or bilirubin levels.
Local: irritation, phlebitis, necrosis with extravasation.

Special considerations

- Give by slow I.V. infusion. In animal studies, rapid I.V. injection has caused seizures.
- Use care to avoid extravasation. Severe irritation and necrosis can result.
- Myelosuppression, which can be severe and cumulative, is dose-limiting.
- Administer by I.V. infusion at a maximum concentration of 1 mg/ml. Incidence of phlebitis increases with higher concentrations.
- Reconstitute with 2.5 ml sterile water for injection to yield a 20 mg/ml solution. Further dilute with dextrose 5% in water or 0.9% sodium chloride injection.
- Avoid mixing with drugs that have a high pH, such as sodium bicarbonate, furosemide, or dexamethasone, to prevent precipitation.

prednimustine (Leo 1031, NSC-134087)
Mostarinia, Sterecyt

How supplied

Tablets: 20 mg

Indications, route, and dosage

Chronic lymphocytic leukemia; non-Hodgkin's lymphoma; ovarian, breast, and prostate cancers
Adults: 20 to 30 mg P.O. daily in one or two divided doses; or 100 to 160 mg/m² P.O. daily for 3 to 5 days, repeated q 10 days to 2 weeks.

Pharmacodynamics

Prednimustine is the prednisolone ester of chlorambucil.

Pharmacokinetics

Absorption: Although prednimustine is administered orally, its absorption is poor.
Excretion: Up to 50% of prednimustine is excreted unchanged in the feces.

Adverse reactions

CNS: confusion, euphoria.
CV: hypertension, edema.
DERM: alopecia (mild), rash, urticaria.
GI: nausea, vomiting (mild), diarrhea, gastritis.
HEMA: *leukopenia, thrombocytopenia.*
Other: fever.

Special considerations

- Hematologic toxicity may be dose-limiting.
- Some clinicians suggest that prednimustine is merely a prodrug of chlorambucil, and that better plasma levels and alkylating activity may be achieved by administering chlorambucil and prednimustine separately.

sodium suramin (antrypol, naganol, NSC-34936)
Suramin

How supplied

Available under investigational protocols from the National Cancer Institute

---

Injection: 1 g/vial (lyophilized powder)

Indications, route, and dosage

Prostate cancer
Men: 350 mg/m^2 daily by continuous I.V. infusion. Drug is usually given until plasma suramin level reaches 250 to 300 mcg/ml. Repeat course of treatment every 2 months.

Pharmacodynamics

Suramin is used to treat early stages of African trypanosomiasis. It is a glycosaminoglycan (GAG) agonist-antagonist, and may inhibit the growth of neoplasms by binding to growth factors such as transforming growth factor beta, platelet-derived growth factor, epidermal growth factor, and basic fibroblast growth factor. Other actions include inhibition of GAG catabolism, DNA polymerase, and growth-regulatory proteins such as transferrin.

Pharmacokinetics

Distribution: Sodium suramin is highly bound to plasma proteins (99%).
Excretion: Most of sodium suramin is excreted in the urine. Elimination half-life is 40 to 50 days.

Adverse reactions

CNS: malaise, paresthesias (perioral and peripheral), progressive muscle weakness, paralysis.
DERM: erythematous rash, urticaria, pruritus.
EENT: vortex keratopathy, with visual disturbances, lacrimation, and photophobia.
GI: bad taste in mouth, nausea, vomiting, constipation.
GU: proteinuria, decreased creatinine clearance, hematuria.
HEMA: *leukopenia, thrombocytopenia;* prolonged prothrombin, thrombin, and partial thromboplastin times; hemorrhage; anemia.
Metabolic: adrenal insufficiency, elevated hepatic enzyme levels, elevated serum creatinine levels, hypocalcemia.
Other: fever.

Special considerations

- Progressive muscle weakness and paralysis are associated with elevated serum levels (380 mcg/ml or more).
- Reconstitute with 10 ml of sterile water to yield a final concentration of 100 mg/ml. Further dilute to a final concentration of 2 to 10 mg/ml with dextrose 5% in water or 0.9% sodium chloride injection.

sparfosate sodium (sparfosic acid, PALA disodium, NSC-224131)

How supplied

Available under investigational protocols from the National Cancer Institute
Injection: 100 mg/ml

Indications, route, and dosage

To enhance the action of fluorouracil in the treatment of various cancers
Adults: 250 mg/m^2 I.V. push weekly with fluorouracil.

Pharmacodynamics

Sparfosate sodium blocks the first step of pyrimidine synthesis by inhibiting the enzyme aspartate transcarbamylase. Use of the drug results in the depletion of cellular pyrimidines, which results in enhanced uptake of fluorouracil into nucleic acids.

Pharmacokinetics

Absorption: Sparfosate is poorly absorbed after oral administration.
Distribution: Sparfosate distributes widely after I.V. injection, with CSF levels ranging from 20% to 40% of concurrent plasma levels 8 hours after injection.
Excretion: About 85% of the drug is excreted unchanged in the urine. Elimination half-life is about 5 hours.

Adverse reactions

CNS: ataxia, lethargy, paresthesias, *seizures*, somnolence.
DERM: rash, flare reactions in previously irradiated areas.
EENT: corneal ulceration, keratoconjunctivitis.
GI: diarrhea, nausea, vomiting, anorexia, mucositis.
HEMA: anemia, *leukopenia*, thrombocytopenia.
Other: fever, phlebitis.

Special considerations

- Skin rash often appears as erythematous or maculopapular, and involves the chest, face, back, and areas of skin folds.
- Although the drug is usually given by I.V. push, it may be infused over 30 minutes as a 1 mg/ml solution. Dilute with 0.9% sodium chloride injection or dextrose 5% in water.
- Solutions are stable for 14 days at room temperature.

taxotere (NSC-628503)

How supplied

Injection: 80 mg/vial

Indications, route, and dosage

Ovarian, breast, and lung cancers

Adults: Several protocols have been tested, including 80 to 100 mg/m² I.V. infused over 6 hours q 3 weeks; 12 mg/m² I.V. infused over 1 hour daily for 5 days, repeated q 3 weeks; 100 mg/m² I.V. infused over 1 hour once weekly for 2 weeks, repeated q 3 weeks; or 90 mg/m² I.V. infused over 24 hours q 3 weeks.

Pharmacodynamics

Taxotere is a semisynthetic derivative of paclitaxel that stabilizes microtubules by inhibiting depolymerization.

Pharmacokinetics

Excretion: Elimination is triphasic, with a terminal elimination half-life of about 12 hours. Less than 5% of a dose appears in the urine.

Adverse reactions

DERM: alopecia, rash.
GI: nausea, vomiting, diarrhea, mucositis.
HEMA: *neutropenia*, thrombocytopenia.

Special considerations

- Taxotere is usually administered by I.V. infusion in dextrose 5% in water or 0.9% sodium chloride injection.
- Hypersensitivity reactions appear as common as those to paclitaxel, but are much less severe.
- Neutropenia is dose-dependent, cumulative, and reversible.
- Skin reactions, including alopecia, occur at doses over 70 mg/m^2.

topotecan (NSC-609699)

How supplied

Available under investigational protocols from the National Cancer Institute
Injection: 5 ml/vial

Indications, route, and dosage

Refractory solid tumors
Adults: 1.3 to 1.6 mg/m^2 I.V. q 3 to 4 weeks. Alternatively, 1.5 mg/m^2 by I.V. infusion for 5 days q 3 to 4 weeks; or 0.65 mg/m^2 by slow I.V. infusion for 5 days q 3 to 4 weeks.

Pharmacodynamics

Topotecan inhibits topoisomerase I, an enzyme that catalyzes the relaxation of supercoiled DNA, an early step in DNA replication.

Pharmacokinetics

Excretion: Elimination half-life is about 3 hours, with 22% to 45% of the drug eliminated unchanged in the urine.

Adverse reactions

CNS: fatigue, malaise, headache, dizziness, light-headedness, peripheral neuropathy, Horner's syndrome.
CV: tachycardia, hypertension.
DERM: rash, acne, fever blisters.
HEMA: *leukopenia, thrombocytopenia, anemia.*
GI: nausea, vomiting, diarrhea.
GU: hematuria.
Metabolic: elevated alkaline phosphatase, AST (formerly SGOT), and creatinine levels; hyperbilirubinemia.
Respiratory: dyspnea.
Other: fever, weight loss, alopecia.

Special considerations

Add 2 ml sterile water to the 5-mg vial to make a 2.5 mg/ml solution. Dilute with 0.9% sodium chloride injection or dextrose 5% in water to a final concentration of 20 to 100 mcg/ml. Drug is stable for 48 hours at room temperature after dilution.

toremifene citrate

How supplied

Available under investigational protocols from Adria Laboratories
Tablets: 10 mg, 20 mg, 60 mg, 200 mg

Indications, route, and dosage

Advanced breast cancer
Women: 60 to 200 mg P.O. daily.

Pharmacodynamics

Toremifene is a nonsteroidal antiestrogen with properties similar to those of tamoxifen. The drug probably also has

---

some antitumor effects independent from estrogen receptor binding because antitumor activity is evident in estrogen receptor-negative cells.

Pharmacokinetics

Absorption: Toremifene is rapidly absorbed after oral administration, with peak plasma levels occurring within 4 hours. Drug is highly bound to plasma proteins.
Metabolism: At least two active metabolites have been identified.
Excretion: Elimination is biphasic, with a terminal elimination half-life of 5 to 6 days.

Adverse reactions

CNS: dizziness, vertigo, lethargy, fatigue, headache, insomnia, tremulousness.
DERM: urticaria.
EENT: eye dryness, cataracts.
GI: nausea, vomiting, abdominal pain.
GU: vaginal discharge, vaginal bleeding.
Respiratory: *pulmonary embolism* (rare).
Metabolic: hypercalcemia, mildly reduced levels of antithrombin III.
Other: hot flashes, sweating, decreased erythrocyte sedimentation rate.

Special considerations

- Toremifene is classified as an estrogen antagonist.
- Preliminary studies suggest that toremifene is tumoristatic rather than tumoricidal.
- Nausea and hot flashes were the most common adverse effects seen in early clinical trials.
- Toremifene is usually administered as a single daily dose.

vindesine sulfate
Eldisine

How supplied

Injection: 5-mg vials

Indications, route, and dosage

Acute lymphoblastic leukemia, breast cancer, malignant melanoma, lymphosarcoma, non-small-cell lung carcinoma

Adults: 3 to 4 mg/m^2 I.V. q 7 to 14 days, or continuous I.V. infusion of 1.2 to 1.5 mg/m^2 daily for 5 days q 3 weeks.

Pharmacodynamics

An antineoplastic agent derived from the vinca alkaloid vinblastine, vindesine arrests mitosis in metaphase by binding to microtubular proteins.

Pharmacokinetics

Absorption: Vindesine is not reliably absorbed from the GI tract; it must be administered I.V.
Distribution: Vindesine is rapidly distributed throughout body tissues.
Metabolism: Metabolism of vindesine occurs in the liver.
Excretion: Vindesine is excreted in the urine and feces.

Adverse reactions

CNS: paresthesias, decreased deep tendon reflex, muscle weakness.
GI: constipation, abdominal cramping, nausea, vomiting.
HEMA: *leukopenia, thrombocytopenia.*
Local: phlebitis, necrosis on extravasation.
Other: *acute bronchospasm,* reversible alopecia, jaw pain, fever with continuous infusions.

Special considerations

- Do not give as a continuous infusion unless patient has a central venous line.
- Avoid extravasation. Vindesine is a painful vesicant. Flush the I.V. line with 10 ml of 0.9% sodium chloride solution beforehand to test vein patency and afterward to flush tubing.
- When reconstituted with the 10-ml diluent provided or 0.9% sodium chloride solution, vindesine is stable for 30 days under refrigeration.
- Do not mix vindesine with other drugs; compatibility with other drugs has not yet been determined.

---

*Canada only   †Off-label use   Italicized adverse reactions are life-threatening.

- After administering, monitor for life-threatening acute bronchospasm, which is most likely to occur in a patient who is also receiving mitomycin.
- To prevent paralytic ileus, encourage patient to drink fluids, increase ambulation, and use stool softeners.
- Assess for depression of Achilles tendon reflex, footdrop or wrist-drop, and slapping gait (late signs of neurotoxicity).
- To detect neuropathy, record patient signatures before each course of therapy and observe for deterioration of handwriting.
- Monitor CBC.

Information for the patient

Instruct patient to report any symptoms of neurotoxicity: numbness and tingling of extremities, jaw pain, constipation (may be an early symptom).

vinorelbine ditartrate (3′,4′-didehydro-4′-deoxy-8′norvincaleukoblastine, NVB)
Navelbine

How supplied

Available under investigational protocols from Burroughs Wellcome
Injection: 10 mg/ml in 10-mg ampules and 50-mg vials
Capsules: 10 mg, 40 mg

Indications, route, and dosage

Non-small-cell lung carcinoma, breast cancer

Adults: 25 to 30 mg/m^2 I.V. weekly; alternatively, 80 mg/m^2 P.O. weekly (for patients with adequate bone marrow reserve) or 50 mg/m^2 P.O. weekly (for patients with poor bone marrow reserve).

Pharmacodynamics

Vinorelbine is a semisynthetic vinca alkaloid derivative of vinblastine. It causes depolymerization of microtubules, leading to impaired synthesis of mitotic spindles. Cell division ultimately stops in G$_2$ and M phases.

Pharmacokinetics

Metabolism: Vinorelbine is metabolized in the liver. Up to 60% of an oral dose undergoes first-pass hepatic metabolism.
Excretion: Vinorelbine's elimination half-life is about 23 hours.

Adverse reactions

CNS: neurotoxicity, decreased deep tendon reflexes, paresthesias.
CV: chest pain, *MI*.
DERM: alopecia.
GI: nausea, vomiting.
HEMA: *neutropenia, leukopenia, thrombocytopenia,* anemia.
Respiratory: dyspnea, pulmonary infiltrates.
Local: phlebitis, tissue necrosis with extravasation.
Other: tumor pain, jaw pain.

Special considerations

- Vinorelbine is classified as a semisynthetic vinca alkaloid.
- Vinorelbine is a vesicant. Use care to avoid extravasation. Minimize risk by diluting the drug in at least 100 ml of 0.9% sodium chloride injection or dextrose 5% in water (D₅W). Give by slow I.V. push or infusion over at least 20 minutes, and follow with a 200- to 300-ml flush with 0.9% sodium chloride injection or D₅W.
- Oral doses should be given on an empty stomach as a single dose.

Pharmacologic management of adverse reactions

Because chemotherapy nonselectively destroys both neoplastic and normal cells, it may adversely affect all of the patient's body systems. In some cases, health care professionals can do little but provide support; in others, drug therapy can help. This chapter explores those adverse reactions to cancer chemotherapy that can be pharmacologically managed—in particular, emesis, stomatitis, and extravasation injury.

CHEMOTHERAPY-INDUCED EMESIS

Emesis is usually related temporally to drug administration, most often occurring within 6 hours of administering chemotherapy; delayed emesis also may occur 2 to 5 days later. Cisplatin, dacarbazine, mechlorethamine, and streptozocin have the highest emesis potential. To determine the emesis potential of various chemotherapeutic drugs, see *Emesis potential of chemotherapeutic drugs,* page 276.

Antiemetics administered prophylactically before the patient's first dose of a chemotherapeutic drug can help prevent emesis. However, studies have shown that patients who've experienced emesis with previous chemotherapy regimens tend to respond poorly to subsequent courses of the same chemotherapy regimen, even when antiemetics are given. This effect may be psychological;

Emesis potential of chemotherapeutic drugs

Very high	High	Moderate	Low
cisplatin	carboplatin	altretamine	bleomycin
cytarabine	carmustine	amsacrine	busulfan
dacarbazine	cyclophospha-	asparaginase	chlorambucil
mechlorethamine	mide	azacitidine	floxuridine
streptozocin	dactinomycin	etoposide	fludarabine
	daunorubicin	idarubicin	fluorouracil
	doxorubicin	ifosfamide	hydroxyurea
	lomustine	mitomycin	melphalan
		mitoxantrone	mercaptopurine
		pentostatin	methotrexate
		plicamycin	paclitaxel
		procarbazine	thioguanine
			thiotepa
			vinblastine
			vincristine

the patient may have learned to associate emesis with chemotherapy.

Before beginning antiemetic therapy, the doctor must ensure that the chemotherapy is causing the emesis. Other causes of emesis include adhesions from previous abdominal surgery, inactivity, metabolic changes, decreased bowel motility with obstruction, constipation or fecal impaction from opioid analgesic therapy, or metastatic brain lesions.

Antiemetic classification

Commonly used antiemetics are classified into eight groups:
• anticholinergics
• antihistamines
• benzodiazepines
• cannabinoids
• corticosteroids
• dopamine antagonists (includes butyrophenones and phenothiazines)

- serotonin antagonists
- miscellaneous agents. For specific dosage information and special considerations related to these agents, see *Antiemetic agents,* pages 278 to 284.

Pharmacology of antiemetics

The most effective antiemetics act in the CNS on a region known as the chemoreceptor trigger zone (CTZ), a specialized area of sensory neurons. Although the CTZ is located in the CNS, its blood flow is not restricted by the blood-brain barrier; this may enhance the ability of the CTZ to react to substances in the blood.

Anticholinergics or antihistamines may be used in combination with dopamine antagonists to control extrapyramidal adverse effects. Used alone, these agents have limited antiemetic impact.

Benzodiazepines act on the CNS, either on cortical pathways or directly on the CTZ, to suppress emesis. Perhaps their most important benefit is the amnesia they produce, which may prevent or eliminate a conditioned response to emesis-producing drugs.

Although their mechanism of action is unknown, cannabinoids probably act on cortical sites as well as on the CTZ. Some clinicians have found these agents to be more effective in patients with a history of marijuana use; their potency is increased when administered with prochlorperazine. A high incidence of adverse CNS reactions, including hallucinations, limits their usefulness, however.

Corticosteroids, such as dexamethasone, offer good antiemetic activity with little toxicity. Their mechanism of action is unknown.

Both dopamine- and serotonin-containing neurons mediate neurotransmission in the CTZ. Antiemetics that block these receptors comprise two of the eight antiemetic drug classes. Phenothiazines and butyrophenones primarily block dopamine receptors; metoclopramide blocks serotonin receptors in high doses.

Other agents act on peripheral neurons, preventing impulses from reaching the CTZ and thus blocking the

(Text continues on page 285.)

Antiemetic agents

ANTICHOLINERGICS

scopolamine (Transderm Scōp)

Dosage
—*Adults:* 1 patch applied behind the ear at least 4 hr before antiemetic effect is required.

Special considerations
• Scopolamine is mostly used to prevent motion sickness; not typically used as a single agent in suppressing chemotherapy-induced emesis.
• Warn patient about proper handling of the patch.
• Tell patient to wash hands after handling patch to avoid getting drug in the eyes.

ANTIHISTAMINES

diphenhydramine (Benadryl)

Dosage
—*Adults:* 25 to 50 mg P.O. q 4 to 6 hr p.r.n.; or 10 mg I.M. or I.V. initially, then 20 to 50 mg I.M. or I.V. q 3 hr p.r.n.
—*Children:* 1 to 1.5 mg/kg P.O. q 4 to 6 hr p.r.n.; or 1 to 1.5 mg/kg I.M. q 6 hr, not to exceed 300 mg/day.

Special considerations
• Protect injectable and elixir solutions from light.
• Elderly patients are usually more sensitive than younger patients to adverse reactions of antihistamines and are likely to experience dizziness, sedation, hyperexcitability, dry mouth, and urine retention.
• Infants and children, especially those under age 6, may exhibit paradoxical hyperexcitability.
• Diphenhydramine may be used to counteract the extrapyramidal effects of high-dose metoclopramide.

BENZODIAZEPINES

lorazepam (Apo-Lorazepam*, Ativan, Novolorazem*)

Dosage
—*Adults:* 2 to 4 mg I.M. or I.V.

Special considerations
• Use as an antiemetic is considered an off-label indication.

*Canada only

Antiemetic agents *(continued)*

BENZODIAZEPINES *(continued)*

lorazepam *(continued)*

• For I.V. administration, dilute lorazepam with an equal volume of a compatible diluent, such as dextrose 5% in water (D$_5$W), sterile water for injection, or 0.9% sodium chloride solution.

• Lorazepam may be injected directly into a vein or into the tubing of a compatible I.V. infusion, such as 0.9% sodium chloride solution or D$_5$W. The rate of lorazepam I.V. injection should not exceed 2 mg/min. Keep emergency resuscitation equipment available when administering I.V.

• Administer diluted lorazepam solutions immediately.

• Do not use discolored or cloudy solutions.

• Administer I.M. dose undiluted, deep into a large muscle mass.

• Advise patient of possible retrograde amnesia after I.V. or I.M. use.

• Parenteral administration is more likely to cause adverse reactions in elderly patients.

CANNABINOIDS

dronabinol (tetrahydrocannabinol, THC) (Marinol)

Dosage

—*Adults and children:* 5 mg/m^2 P.O. 1 to 3 hr before administration of chemotherapy; then give same dose q 2 to 4 hr after chemotherapy for a total of four to six doses daily. Dose may be increased in increments of 2.5 mg/m^2 to a maximum of 15 mg/m^2 per dose.

Special considerations

• Dronabinol is the major active ingredient of *Cannabis sativa* (marijuana) and therefore has a potential for abuse.

• Warn patient to avoid driving and other activities requiring sound judgment until extent of CNS depressant effects are known.

• Urge family to ensure that patient is supervised during and immediately after treatment.

• Caution patient and family to anticipate drug's mood-altering effects.

CORTICOSTEROIDS

dexamethasone (Decadron, Hexadrol)

Dosage

—*Adults:* 10 to 20 mg P.O. daily.

(continued)

Antiemetic agents *(continued)*

CORTICOSTEROIDS *(continued)*

dexamethasone *(continued)*

Special considerations
• Use as an antiemetic is considered an off-label indication.
• Dexamethasone is contraindicated in patients with systemic fungal infections and for alternate-day therapy; also contraindicated in patients with hypersensitivity to any component of the drug.
• Use cautiously in patients with GI ulceration or renal disease, hypertension, osteoporosis, varicella, vaccinia, exanthema, diabetes mellitus, Cushing's syndrome, thromboembolic disorders, seizures, myasthenia gravis, metastatic cancer, CHF, tuberculosis, ocular herpes simplex, hypoalbuminemia, emotional instability, or psychotic tendencies; also use cautiously in children.
• Monitor serum potassium levels.
• Give oral dose with food when possible.

DOPAMINE ANTAGONISTS: BUTYROPHENONES

droperidol (Inapsine)

Dosage
—Adults: 6.25 mg I.M. or by slow I.V. injection.

Special considerations
• Use cautiously in patients with hypotension and other cardiovascular diseases; also use cautiously in patients taking such CNS depressants as alcohol, opiates, and sedatives because droperidol may potentiate the effects of these drugs.
• Monitor vital signs and watch carefully for extrapyramidal reactions.
• Droperidol may potentiate the respiratory and CNS depressant effects of opiate analgesics; use together cautiously.

haloperidol (Haldol)

Dosage
—*Adults:* 0.5 to 5 mg P.O. b.i.d. or t.i.d., increased p.r.n.

Special considerations
• Use as an antiemetic is considered an off-label indication.
• Protect drug from light. Slight yellowing of oral concentrate is common; this does not affect drug potency. Discard markedly discolored solutions.

Antiemetic agents (continued)

DOPAMINE ANTAGONISTS: BUTYROPHENONES (continued)

haloperidol (continued)

• Warn patient against activities that require alertness and good psychomotor coordination until CNS response to drug is determined.
• Advise patient to report adverse reactions, such as extrapyramidal reactions.
• Haloperidol is not recommended for children under age 3. Children are especially prone to extrapyramidal adverse reactions.

DOPAMINE ANTAGONISTS: PHENOTHIAZINES

prochlorperazine (Compazine, Stemetil*)
prochlorperazine edisylate (Compazine)
prochlorperazine maleate (Chlorazine, Compazine, Compazine Spansule, Stemetil*)

Dosage
—*Adults:* 5 to 10 mg P.O. t.i.d. or q.i.d., 15 mg of sustained-release form P.O. on arising, or 10 mg of sustained-release form P.O. q 12 hr; 25 mg rectally b.i.d.; or 5 to 10 mg I.M. injected deeply into upper outer quadrant of gluteal region. Repeat q 3 to 4 hr, p.r.n. May be given I.V. Maximum parenteral dosage is 40 mg daily.
—*Children weighing 18 to 39 kg:* 2.5 mg P.O. or rectally t.i.d. or 5 mg P.O. or rectally b.i.d., or, 0.132 mg/kg deep I.M. injection. (Control typically is obtained with one dose.) Maximum dosage is 15 mg daily.
—*Children weighing 14 to 17 kg:* 2.5 mg P.O. or rectally b.i.d. or t.i.d., or 0.132 mg/kg deep I.M. injection. (Control typically is obtained with one dose.) Maximum dosage is 10 mg daily.
—*Children weighing 9 to 13 kg:* 2.5 mg P.O. or rectally daily or b.i.d., or 0.132 mg/kg deep I.M. injection. (Control typically is obtained with one dose.) Maximum dosage is 7.5 mg daily.

Special considerations
• Prochlorperazine is contraindicated in patients with blood dyscrasias and bone marrow depression; it should not be used with adrenergic-blocking agents or spinal or epidural anesthetics.
• Concomitant use with such sympathomimetics as epinephrine may cause epinephrine reversal (hypotensive response to epinephrine).

(continued)

*Canada only

Antiemetic agents (continued)

DOPAMINE ANTAGONISTS: PHENOTHIAZINES (continued)

prochlorperazine
prochlorperazine edisylate
prochlorperazine maleate (continued)

• Prochlorperazine may discolor urine.
• Tell patient to avoid spilling the liquid form. Skin contact may cause irritation. Injectable formulation may also cause a rash after contact with skin.

SEROTONIN ANTAGONISTS

metoclopramide hydrochloride (Reglan)

Dosage
—*Adults:* 2 mg/kg I.V. q 2 hr for five doses, beginning 30 min before emetogenic chemotherapy.

Special considerations
• Metoclopramide is contraindicated in patients with known hypersensitivity to the drug or to sulfonamides.
• Use cautiously in children because they may have a higher incidence of adverse CNS reactions and in patients with a history of breast cancer because metoclopramide stimulates prolactin secretion.
• For I.V. push administration, use undiluted and inject over a 1- to 2-min period. For I.V. infusion, dilute with 50 ml of dextrose 5% in water, dextrose 5% in 0.45% sodium chloride solution, 0.9% sodium chloride injection, or lactated Ringer's injection, and infuse over at least 15 min.
• Diphenhydramine may be used to counteract the extrapyramidal effects of high-dose metoclopramide.
• Warn patient to avoid driving for at least 2 hr after each dose because drug may cause drowsiness.
• Tell patient to report any extrapyramidal reactions and to avoid alcohol.

ondansetron hydrochloride (Zofran)

Dosage
—*Adults and children over age 12:* 8 mg P.O. 30 min before chemotherapy begins. Follow with 8 mg P.O. 4 hr and 8 hr after the first dose. Then follow with 8 mg P.O. q 8 hr for 1 to 2 days. Alternatively, administer a single dose of 32 mg I.V. infused over 15 min beginning 30 min before

Antiemetic agents *(continued)*

SEROTONIN ANTAGONISTS *(continued)*

ondansetron hydrochloride *(continued)*

chemotherapy; or administer in three doses of 0.15 mg/kg I.V. Give first dose 30 min before chemotherapy; administer subsequent doses 4 and 8 hr after the first dose. Infuse drug over 15 min.
—*Children age 4 to 11:* 4 mg P.O. 30 min before chemotherapy begins. Follow with 4 mg P.O. 4 hr and 8 hr after the first dose. Then follow with 4 mg P.O. q 8 hr for 1 to 2 days. Alternatively, administer a single dose of 32 mg I.V. over 15 min, beginning 30 min before chemotherapy; administer subsequent doses 4 and 8 hr after the first dose. Infuse drug over 15 min.

Special considerations
• Use cautiously in patients with hepatic failure. Limit daily dosage (oral or I.V.) to 8 mg.
• For I.V. use, dilute the drug in 50 ml of dextrose 5% in water injection or 0.9% sodium chloride injection before administration. The drug is also stable for up to 48 hr after dilution in 5% dextrose in 0.9% sodium chloride injection, 5% dextrose in 0.45%, sodium chloride injection, and 3% sodium chloride injection.

MISCELLANEOUS AGENTS

benzquinamide hydrochloride (Emete-Con)

Dosage
—*Adults:* 25 mg I.V. slowly (1 mg/min) or 50 mg I.M., repeated in 1 hr, then q 3 to 4 hr.

Special considerations
• Blood pressure changes and arrhythmias are more likely to occur with I.V. use.
• Give I.M. injection into a large muscle mass; use deltoid muscle only if well developed. Be careful to avoid inadvertent I.V. injection.

chlorpromazine hydrochloride (Novo-Chlorpromazine*, Thorazine)

Dosage
—*Adults:* 10 to 25 mg P.O. or I.M. q 4 to 6 hr, p.r.n.; or 50 to 100 mg rectally q 6 to 8 hr, p.r.n.

(continued)

Antiemetic agents (continued)

MISCELLANEOUS AGENTS (continued)

chlorpromazine hydrochloride (continued)

—*Children:* 0.25 mg/kg P.O. q 4 to 6 hr; or 0.25 mg/kg I.M. q 6 to 8 hr; or 0.5 mg/kg rectally q 6 to 8 hr.

Special considerations
• Contraindicated in CNS depression, bone marrow suppression, subcortical damage, Reye's syndrome, and coma; also contraindicated with use of spinal or epidural anesthetic, or adrenergic blocking agents.
• Use parenteral form cautiously in asthmatics and in patients allergic to sulfites.
• Acute dystonic reactions may be treated with I.V. diphenhydramine.
• Tell patient that the drug may discolor the urine.
• Give deep I.M. only in upper outer quadrant of buttocks. Massage slowly afterward to prevent sterile abscess. Injection stings.
• Liquid (oral) and parenteral forms of drug can cause contact dermatitis. If susceptible, wear gloves when preparing solutions of this drug, and prevent contact with skin and clothing.

thiethylperazine maleate (Norzine, Torecan*)

Dosage
—*Adults:* 10 mg P.O., I.M., or rectally daily, b.i.d., or t.i.d.

Special considerations
• Contraindicated in severe CNS depression, hepatic disease, coma, phenothiazine hypersensitivity.
• Don't give I.V. May cause severe hypotension.
• Warn patient about hypotension. Advise him to stay in bed for 1 hr after receiving the drug.
• If drug gets on skin, wash off at once to prevent contact dermatitis.

trimethobenzamide hydrochloride (Tigan)

Dosage
—*Adults:* 250 mg P.O. t.i.d. or q.i.d., or 200 mg I.M. t.i.d. or q.i.d.

Special considerations
• Give I.M. injection deep into the upper outer quadrant of the buttock to minimize pain and local irritation.

---

*Canada only

vomiting reflex. Ondansetron, a specific serotonin 5-HT$_3$ receptor antagonist, blocks the 5-HT$_3$ receptors on the GI tract's vagal afferent nerve terminals. Blocking these receptors may decrease the transmission of stimulatory impulses from the periphery to the vomiting center.

Miscellaneous agents, including trimethobenzamide and benzquinamide, have less antiemetic efficacy. They probably act directly on the CTZ.

Overview of adverse reactions to antiemetics
The most common adverse reactions associated with anticholinergic antiemetics are dry mouth, tachycardia, dysuria, urine retention, and constipation, which reflect the drugs' pharmacologic effects. In higher dosages, blurred vision, tinnitus, or CNS disturbances may occur.

Most adverse reactions to antihistamine antiemetics are predictable, mild, and easy to control. Although all such drugs produce some drowsiness, reducing the dose may decrease drowsiness without compromising the antiemetic effect. Children are more prone to paradoxical CNS stimulation than adults, with signs ranging from restlessness, insomnia, and euphoria to tremor and even seizures. Other adverse CNS reactions include dizziness, headache, and lassitude. Administering these drugs with food or milk may decrease the mild nausea or epigastric distress associated with them. Anorexia that lasts for several weeks may also result from long-term administration of antihistamine antiemetics.

Benzodiazepines can cause confusion, depression, drowsiness, lethargy, ataxia, dizziness, nightmares, fatigue, and a hangover effect. The amnesia that benzodiazepines can induce may help patients receiving chemotherapeutic drugs with high emesis potential. Rarely, bradycardia or transient hypotension occurs with parenteral administration.

Cannabinoids commonly cause dizziness, ataxia, disorientation, memory lapse, and muddled thinking. Some patients may develop paranoia, perceptual difficulties, hallucinations, headache, dry mouth, tachycardia, and orthostatic hypotension.

Short-term courses of corticosteroid therapy rarely produce adverse reactions. Although adverse CNS reactions such as euphoria, insomnia, headache, nervousness, restlessness, or mental changes may occur with short-term, high-dose therapy, toxic signs and symptoms rarely occur when corticosteroid antiemetics are used for less than 3 weeks, even at high dosages. Chronic use of corticosteroids causes adverse physiologic reactions, including suppression of the hypothalamic-pituitary-adrenal (HPA) axis, cushingoid appearance, muscle weakness, and osteoporosis.

Adverse CNS reactions are a major problem for patients receiving dopamine antagonist antiemetics. Mild-to-moderate sedation occurs in 50% to 80% of patients; chlorpromazine, a phenothiazine, produces the greatest incidence. Tolerance to the sedative effect typically develops over several days of therapy. Confusion may also occur, especially in elderly patients. Other adverse CNS reactions to dopamine antagonist antiemetics include anxiety, euphoria, agitation, depression, headache, insomnia, restlessness, and weakness. These drugs also may lower the seizure threshold and should be used cautiously in patients predisposed to seizures.

Because they block central dopamine receptors, phenothiazine and butyrophenone antiemetics may produce three types of extrapyramidal reactions: dystonic reactions, feelings of motor restlessness, and parkinsonism. Dystonic reactions and feelings of motor restlessness occur more frequently in children, especially if they are febrile or dehydrated. Signs and symptoms of parkinsonism occur more often in elderly patients, especially those with brain damage.

Persistent dyskinesias, such as tardive dyskinesia, are more likely with prolonged therapy. However, such disorders have surfaced even after relatively short-term, low dosages of dopamine antagonists.

Phenothiazine antiemetics may also cause hypotension and orthostatic hypotension with tachycardia, syncope, and dizziness. Chlorpromazine produces the highest incidence of hypotensive effects; prochlorperazine and thiethylperazine, the lowest. Tolerance to hypotensive effects typically develops over time.

Although hypersensitivity reactions can result when phenothiazines are used as antipsychotics, such reactions rarely occur when they are used as antiemetics. However, cholestatic jaundice, blood dyscrasias, dermatologic reactions, photosensitivity, and other hypersensitivity reactions have occurred within the first few months of phenothiazine therapy. Granulocytopenia, the most commonly reported adverse hematologic reaction, is also rare. Phenothiazines produce many dermatologic effects, especially with long-term therapy.

Serotonin antagonists, such as ondansetron, generally are well tolerated. Their most common adverse reaction is headache; other effects, such as akathisia, acute dystonic reactions, and generalized seizures, are rare. Adverse anticholinergic reactions typically include dry mouth, blurred vision, constipation, and urine retention.

The most common adverse reactions seen with miscellaneous agents involve the CNS. Benzquinamide may cause drowsiness, restlessness, or fatigue. Trimethobenzamide may produce extrapyramidal reactions, such as acute dystonia and dyskinesia; if these occur, discontinue the drug. Hypersensitivity reactions, manifested by rashes and photosensitivity, may occur. Blood dyscrasias (including granulocytopenia, hemolytic anemia, leukopenia, thrombocytopenia, and pancytopenia) have occurred rarely.

Combination therapy

Although serotonin antagonists, such as ondansetron, have improved treatment of acute emesis, some evidence suggests other drugs are more effective in treating delayed emesis. Comparison trials have found that ondansetron is significantly superior to metoclopramide in treating emesis in the first 2 days following chemotherapy. Thereafter, metoclopramide is equally effective or superior to ondansetron.

Combination protocols for antiemetic therapy

Antiemetic efficacy can be enhanced when certain drugs are administered in combination. The following chart is a sample of representative combination protocols used with emetogenic chemotherapy.

ondansetron	32 mg I.V. infused over 15 min beginning 30 min before chemotherapy
dexamethasone	10 mg I.V.
lorazepam	1 to 1.5 mg/m^2 I.V.
metoclopramide	2 mg/kg I.V. q 2 to 4 hr for 3 doses
dexamethasone	10 mg I.V.
lorazepam	1 to 1.5 mg/m^2 I.V.
diphenhydramine	20 to 50 mg I.V. q 6 to 8 hr

Some researchers have determined that combination therapy is more effective than single drug therapy in managing chemotherapy-induced emesis. For examples of combinations, see *Combination protocols for antiemetic therapy.*

Supportive care

It's critical to help the chemotherapy patient manage nausea and vomiting. Patients who can't tolerate these adverse effects may refuse treatment. Establishing an antiemetic therapy plan with the first dose of chemotherapy can avoid the anticipatory emesis some patients experience before subsequent doses.

To ensure optimal effects and avoid complications, follow these guidelines:

- Encourage the patient to express anxious feelings.
- Provide a pleasant, quiet environment during drug administration.
- Encourage the patient to listen to music or engage in relaxation exercises, meditation, or hypnosis to promote feelings of control and well-being.
- Adjust the drug administration schedule to meet the patient's needs, if possible. For example, some patients prefer treatments in the evening when they find sedation comfortable.

- Encourage adequate nutritional and fluid intake, and provide supplements, if needed.
- Assess the patient for dehydration, and monitor weight and serum electrolyte levels.

STOMATITIS

The incidence and severity of stomatitis—a temporary inflammation of the oral mucosa ranging from mild to debilitating—varies with the drug, the dose, and the administration schedule. In some cases, the patient complains of pain before inflammation is visible. For a list of drugs that may cause this reaction, see *Chemotherapeutic drugs that cause stomatitis*, page 290.

Treatment

Advise the patient to brush his teeth frequently (if tolerated) and use mouth rinses routinely. Patients with moderate-to-severe stomatitis find chlorhexidine mouth rinse intolerable because of its high alcohol content; advise such patients to use a solution of 0.2% chlorhexidine gluconate diluted with alcohol-free mouthwash. Rinsing with sucralfate dissolved in alcohol-free mouthwash or using a saliva substitute may also soothe the oral mucosa. Treat pain with local anesthetics (such as viscous lidocaine 2% or dyclonine hydrochloride). Severe pain may require systemic analgesics.

Researchers investigating patients receiving fluorouracil and leucovorin rescue who experience a high incidence of stomatitis have found that those who swished ice chips in their mouth for 5 minutes before treatment and for a total of 30 minutes had a reduced incidence of stomatitis. This easy and inexpensive treatment requires patient cooperation, however.

The patient who develops a secondary fungal infection should receive an antifungal agent, such as nystatin suspension. Left untreated, the infection will spread throughout the GI tract, causing possible ulceration with epigastric distress and diarrhea.

Chemotherapeutic drugs that cause stomatitis

The following drugs are representative of chemotherapeutic drugs that can cause stomatitis. Consult the list below to determine if the particular drug your patient is receiving can cause stomatitis.

High incidence	Common
aldesleukin	fludarabine
bleomycin	interferons
cytarabine	levamisole
dactinomycin	mitomycin
daunorubicin	mercaptopurine
doxorubicin	plicamycin
fluorouracil	thioguanine
leucovorin calcium	vinblastine
methotrexate	vincristine

Prevention

Good oral hygiene is the best prevention for stomatitis. Use the following patient-teaching guidelines to help prevent this adverse effect and make the patient more comfortable:

- Before chemotherapy starts, teach preventive mouth care, including frequent toothbrushing with a soft-bristled brush or a soft sponge, and rinsing with 0.9% sodium chloride solution, baking soda in water, or chlorhexidine gluconate.
- Tell the patient to clean his teeth before and after meals. Warn the patient to floss cautiously.
- Advise frequent warm-water rinses to relieve discomfort or dry mouth.
- Tell the patient to avoid smoking and drinking alcohol, which worsen the condition.
- Warn the patient to avoid hot or cold drinks and spicy or sour foods if ulceration develops.
- Tell the patient or caregiver to notify the doctor if he notices white patches in his mouth.

EXTRAVASATION INJURY

Extravasation, the leakage of a drug into perivascular or subcutaneous spaces during I.V. administration, can be a serious complication of antineoplastic drug administration. The extent and severity of the local tissue injury varies with the drug, its concentration, and the volume leaked into tissues. For information on drugs associated with local tissue injury following extravasation, see *Determining vesicant potential.*

Determining vesicant potential

To administer a chemotherapeutic drug safely, you need to know whether it's a vesicant (producing blisters), an irritant (producing undue sensitivity), or a nonvesicant. Before administering a vesicant, check your facility's policy. Because vein integrity decreases with use, some facilities require that vesicants be administered before other drugs. Others require that vesicants be given after other drugs because vesicants increase vein fragility. Because of the lack of clinical data regarding vesicant potential, investigational drugs are not included here.

Vesicants

- dactinomycin
- daunorubicin
- doxorubicin
- idarubicin
- mechlorethamine
- mitomycin
- vinblastine
- vincristine

Irritants

- bleomycin
- carmustine
- cisplatin
- dacarbazine
- etoposide
- fluorouracil
- mitoxantrone
- paclitaxel
- plicamycin
- streptozocin
- teniposide

Nonvesicants

- asparaginase
- busulfan
- carboplatin
- chlorambucil
- cyclophosphamide
- cytarabine
- floxuridine
- ifosfamide
- melphalan
- methotrexate
- thiotepa
- trimetrexate

Treatment

Because treatment for extravasation injury remains somewhat controversial, each facility should develop standing protocols so that suspected extravasation is treated rapidly. Early recognition and treatment can prevent serious injury. If extravasation occurs, take the following steps:

- Discontinue the infusion.
- Check the facility's policy to determine whether you should remove the needle and withdraw some fluid to remove extravasated drug or leave the needle in place.
- Elevate the extremity and apply ice for 24 to 48 hours, replacing the ice pack every 1 to 2 hours. If the extravasated drug is a vinca alkaloid, such as vinblastine, vincristine, or vindesine, apply heat instead. (For more information, see *Heat vs. cold: How to treat extravasation.*)
- Administer a corticosteroid (such as methylprednisolone sodium succinate 40 to 125 mg, or dexamethasone 4 mg) intradermally and subcutaneously at the site. Start at the site periphery and give multiple injections in a circular fashion, working toward the center. Total dose varies with the extent of injury.

Heat vs. cold: How to treat extravasation

Controversy continues over the use of warm compresses versus cold on the site of extravasation injury. Applying heat causes vasodilation, which increases blood flow to the area, enhances systemic drug absorption, and decreases local toxicity. However, some experts argue that the increased dispersion of a vesicant drug enhances cellular destruction. Moist heat indeed may enhance tissue maceration and necrosis and should be avoided. Heat is indicated, however, for vinca alkaloid extravasation.

Applying cold localizes the drug in the immediate area of the extravasation by promoting vasoconstriction. Cold compresses also decrease local discomfort and irritation. Because of the risk of increased local injury, however, vinca alkaloid extravasation should not be treated with cold compresses.

Antidotes for vesicant extravasation

Although the practice is controversial, some clinicians routinely administer antidotes following the extravasation of vesicant chemotherapeutic drugs. The following table details selected vesicants with their antidotes and mechanisms of action.

Vesicant	Antidote	Mechanisms of action
carmustine	sodium bicarbonate 8.4%	Inactives carmustine
dactinomycin	sodium thiosulfate 10% ascorbic acid 50 mg	Decreases binding of dactinomycin to cellular DNA
daunorubicin	sodium bicarbonate 8.4%	Decreases binding of daunorubicin to cellular DNA
doxorubicin	sodium bicarbonate 8.4%	Decreases binding of doxorubicin to cellular DNA
mechlorethamine	sodium thiosulfate 10%	Inactivates mechlorethamine
mitomycin	sodium thiosulfate 10%	Inactivates mitomycin
vinblastine vincristine	sodium bicarbonate 8.4% hyaluronidase 150 U	Precipitates drug with bicarbonate

- Administer an antidote as appropriate (see *Antidotes for vesicant extravasation*). This is a controversial step because there is a lack of data supporting the safety and efficacy of antidotes. In addition, there is some evidence that sodium bicarbonate, a commonly used antidote, may irritate tissue.
- Apply a corticosteroid cream, such as hydrocortisone 1%, to the site. Cover with a sterile gauze pad.

- Tell the patient to exercise the affected extremity four times daily.
- Obtain a consultation with a plastic surgeon or physical therapist, as appropriate.

Prevention

To safely administer vesicants, use a central line. If a central line is not in place, start an I.V. line in the largest, straightest vein possible, using a new site for each administration. Don't infuse drugs into extremities with impaired circulation or near joints, where sudden flexion is a possibility. To avoid complications, follow these guidelines:

- Warn the patient to avoid moving during drug administration.
- Before administration, check the patency and integrity of the I.V. line.
- Lower the I.V. bag and note blood return.
- Monitor the I.V. site for redness, swelling, pain, or burning. Tell the patient to report these adverse reactions immediately.
- Note any change in the I.V. drip rate caused by the patient's changing position.
- Inject the vesicant drug slowly, using the side arm of a free-flowing I.V. infusion. Ensure vigilant and clear observation of the I.V. site during administration.

Appendices and Index

ABBREVIATIONS

ALT	serum alanine aminotransferase, formerly SGPT
AST	serum aspartate aminotransferase, formerly SGOT
ATP	adenosine triphosphate
AV	atrioventricular
b.i.d.	twice daily
BUN	blood urea nitrogen
cAMP	cyclic 3′, 5′adenosine monophosphate
CBC	complete blood count
CHF	congestive heart failure
CK	creatine kinase
CMV	cytomegalovirus
CNS	central nervous system
COPD	chronic obstructive pulmonary disease
CPR	cardiopulmonary resuscitation
CSF	cerebrospinal fluid
CV	cardiovascular
CVA	cerebrovascular accident
CVP	central venous pressure
DNA	deoxyribonucleic acid
ECG	electrocardiogram
EEG	electroencephalogram
EENT	eyes, ears, nose, throat
FDA	Food and Drug Administration
G	gauge
g	gram
GFR	glomerular filtration rate
GI	gastrointestinal
G6PD	glucose-6-phosphate dehydrogenase
GU	genitourinary
HEMA	hematologic
h.s.	at bedtime
I.M.	intramuscular
IND	investigational new drug
IU	International Unit
I.V.	intravenous
kg	kilogram
L	liter

LDH	lactate dehydrogenase
M	molar
m²	square meter
MAO	monoamine oxidase
mcg	microgram
mEq	milliequivalent
mg	milligram
MI	myocardial infarction
ml	milliliter
mm³	cubic millimeter
ng	nanogram (millimicrogram)
NSAID	nonsteroidal anti-inflammatory drug
P.O.	by mouth
P.R.	by rectum
p.r.n.	as needed
q	every
q.d.	every day
q.i.d.	four times daily
q.o.d.	every other day
RBC	red blood cell
RNA	ribonucleic acid
RSV	respiratory syncytial virus
SA	sinoatrial
S.C.	subcutaneous
SIADH	syndrome of inappropriate antidiuretic hormone
t.i.d.	three times daily
WBC	white blood cell

Cancer chemotherapy: Acronyms and protocols

Combination chemotherapy is well established for treatment of cancer. The chart below lists commonly used acronyms and protocols, including standard dosages for specific cancers.

ACRONYM AND INDICATION	DRUG		DOSAGE
	Generic name	Trade name	
AA (Leukemia— AML, induction)	cytarabine (ara-C)	Cytosar-U	100 mg/m² daily by continuous I.V. infusion for 7 to 10 days
	doxorubicin	Adriamycin	30 mg/m² I.V., days 1 to 3
ABVD (Hodgkin's lymphoma)	doxorubicin	Adriamycin	25 mg/m² I.V., days 1 and 15
	bleomycin	Blenoxane	10 units/m² I.V., days 1 and 15
	vinblastine	Velban	6 mg/m² I.V., days 1 and 15
	dacarbazine	DTIC-Dome	375 mg/m² I.V., days 1 and 15 *Repeat cycle q 28 days.*
AC (Multiple myeloma)	doxorubicin	Adriamycin	30 mg/m² I.V., day 1
	carmustine	BiCNU	30 mg/m² I.V., day 1 *Repeat cycle q 21 to 28 days.*
AC (Bony sarcoma)	doxorubicin	Adriamycin	75 to 90 mg/m² by 96-hour continuous I.V. infusion
	cisplatin	Platinol	90 to 120 mg/m² IA or I.V., day 6 *Repeat cycle q 28 days.*
AFM (Breast cancer)	doxorubicin	Adriamycin	25 mg/m² by continuous I.V. infusion, days 1 to 3
	fluorouracil (5-FU)	Adrucil	400 mg/m² I.V., days 1 to 5
	methotrexate	Folex	250 mg/m² I.V., day 18
	leucovorin calcium	Wellcovorin	15 mg/m² P.O. q 6 hours, days 19 to 20 *Repeat cycle q 21 days for four cycles.*
AP (Ovarian cancer, epithelial)	doxorubicin	Adriamycin	50 to 60 mg/m² I.V., day 1
	cisplatin	Platinol	50 to 60 mg/m² I.V., day 1 *Repeat cycle q 21 days.*
APE (EAP) (Gastric cancer)	doxorubicin	Adriamycin	20 mg/m² I.V. daily, days 1 and 7
	cisplatin	Platinol	40 mg/m² I.V. daily, days 2 and 8
	etoposide (VP-16)	VePesid	120 mg/m² I.V. daily, days 4, 5, and 6 *Repeat cycle q 8 weeks.*

Cancer chemotherapy: Acronyms and protocols *(continued)*

ACRONYM AND INDICATION	DRUG Generic name	DRUG Trade name	DOSAGE
ASHAP (Non-Hodgkin's lymphoma)	doxorubicin	Adriamycin	10 mg/m² daily by continuous I.V. infusion, days 1 to 4
	cisplatin	Platinol	25 mg/m² daily by continuous I.V. infusion days 1 to 4
	cytarabine (ara-C)	Cytosar-U	1,500 mg/m² I.V. immediately after completion of doxorubicin and cisplatin therapy
	methylprednisolone	Solu-Medrol	500 mg I.V. daily, days 1 to 5 *Repeat cycle q 21 to 25 days.*
BACON (Non-small-cell lung cancer)	bleomycin	Blenoxane	30 units I.V. q 6 weeks, day 2
	doxorubicin	Adriamycin	40 mg/m² I.V. q 4 weeks, day 1
	lomustine (CCNU)	CeeNU	65 mg/m² P.O. q 8 weeks, day 1
	vincristine	Oncovin	0.75 to 1 mg/m² I.V. q 6 weeks, day 2
	mechlorethamine (nitrogen mustard)	Mustargen	8 mg/m² I.V. q 4 weeks, day 1
BACOP (Non-Hodgkin's lymphoma)	bleomycin	Blenoxane	5 units/m² I.V. daily, days 15 and 22
	doxorubicin	Adriamycin	25 mg/m² I.V., days 1 and 8
	cyclophosphamide	Cytoxan	650 mg/m² I.V., days 1 and 8
	vincristine	Oncovin	1.4 mg/m² (2 mg maximum) I.V., days 1 and 8
	prednisone	Deltasone	60 mg/m² P.O., days 15 to 28 *Repeat cycle q 28 days.*
BCP (Multiple myeloma)	carmustine	BiCNU	75 mg/m² I.V., day 1
	cyclophosphamide	Cytoxan	400 mg/m² I.V., day 1
	prednisone	Deltasone	75 mg P.O., days 1 to 7 *Repeat cycle q 28 days.*
BEP (Genitourinary cancer)	bleomycin	Blenoxane	30 units I.V., days 2, 9, and 16
	etoposide (VP-16)	VePesid	100 mg/m², days 1 to 5
	cisplatin	Platinol	20 mg/m² I.V., days 1 to 5
BHD (Malignant melanoma)	carmustine	BiCNU	100 to 150 mg/m² I.V. q 6 weeks
	hydroxyurea	Hydrea	1,480 mg/m² P.O. q 3 weeks, days 1 to 5
	dacarbazine	DTIC-Dome	100 to 150 mg/m² I.V. q 3 weeks, days 1 to 5
CA (Breast cancer)	cyclophosphamide	Cytoxan	200 mg/m² P.O., days 3 to 6
	doxorubicin	Adriamycin	40 mg/m² I.V., day 1 *Repeat cycle q 21 to 28 days.*

(continued)

Cancer chemotherapy: Acronyms and protocols *(continued)*

ACRONYM AND INDICATION	DRUG		DOSAGE
	Generic name	Trade name	
CAE (ACE) (Small-cell lung cancer)	cyclophosphamide	Cytoxan	1 g/m² I.V., day 1
	doxorubicin	Adriamycin	50 mg/m² I.V., day 1
	etoposide (VP-16)	VePesid	80 to 120 mg/m² I.V., day 1 *Repeat cycle q 21 days.*
CAF (FAC) (Breast cancer)	cyclophosphamide	Cytoxan	100 mg/m² P.O., days 1 to 14
	doxorubicin	Adriamycin	30 mg/m² I.V., days 1 and 8
	fluorouracil (5-FU)	Adrucil	400 to 500 mg/m² I.V., days 1 and 8 *Repeat cycle q 28 days.*
or	cyclophosphamide	Cytoxan	500 mg/m² I.V., day 1
	doxorubicin	Adriamycin	50 mg/m² I.V., day 1
	fluorouracil (5-FU)	Adrucil	500 mg/m² I.V., day 1 *Repeat cycle q 21 days.*
CAMP (Non-small-cell lung cancer)	cyclophosphamide	Cytoxan	300 mg/m² I.V., days 1 and 8
	doxorubicin	Adriamycin	20 mg/m² I.V., days 1 and 8
	methotrexate sodium	Folex	15 mg/m² I.V., days 1 and 8
	procarbazine	Matulane	100 mg/m² P.O., days 1 to 10 *Repeat cycle q 28 days.*
CAP (Genitourinary cancer)	cisplatin	Platinol	60 mg/m² I.V., day 1
	doxorubicin	Adriamycin	40 mg/m² I.V., day 1
	cyclophosphamide	Cytoxan	400 mg/m² I.V., day 1 *Repeat cycle q 21 days.*
CAP (Non-small-cell lung cancer)	cyclophosphamide	Cytoxan	400 mg/m² I.V., day 1
	doxorubicin	Adriamycin	40 mg/m² I.V., day 1
	cisplatin	Platinol	60 mg/m² I.V., day 1 *Repeat cycle q 28 days.*
CAP (PAC) (Ovarian cancer, epithelial)	cisplatin	Platinol	50 mg/m² I.V., day 1
	doxorubicin	Adriamycin	50 mg/m² I.V., day 1
	cyclophosphamide	Cytoxan	500 mg/m² I.V., day 1 *Repeat cycle q 21 days for eight cycles.*
CAV (Small-cell lung cancer)	cyclophosphamide	Cytoxan	750 mg/m² I.V., day 1
	doxorubicin	Adriamycin	50 mg/m² I.V., day 1
	vincristine	Oncovin	2 mg/m² I.V., day 1 *Repeat cycle q 3 weeks.*

Cancer chemotherapy: Acronyms and protocols *(continued)*

ACRONYM AND INDICATION	DRUG		DOSAGE
	Generic name	Trade name	
CAVe (Hodgkin's lymphoma)	lomustine (CCNU)	CeeNU	100 mg/m² I.V., day 1
	doxorubicin	Adriamycin	60 mg/m² I.V., day 1
	vinblastine	Velban	5 mg/m² I.V., day 1 *Repeat cycle q 6 weeks.*
CC (Ovarian cancer, epithelial)	carboplatin	Paraplatin	300 mg/m² I.V., day 1
	cyclophosphamide	Cytoxan	600 mg/m² I.V., day 1 *Repeat cycle q 20 days.*
CD (DC) (Leukemia— ANLL, consolidation)	cytarabine (ara-C)	Cytosar-U	3,000 mg/m² I.V. q 12 hours for 6 days
	daunorubicin	Cerubidine	30 mg/m² I.V. daily for 3 days, after cytarabine therapy
CDC (Ovarian cancer, epithelial)	carboplatin	Paraplatin	300 mg/m² I.V., day 1
	doxorubicin	Adriamycin	40 mg/m² I.V., day 1
	cyclophosphamide	Cytoxan	500 mg/m² I.V., day 1 *Repeat cycle q 28 days.*
CF (Head and neck cancer)	cisplatin	Platinol	100 mg/m² I.V., day 1
	fluorouracil (5-FU)	Adrucil	1,000 mg/m² daily by continuous I.V. infusion, days 1 to 5 *Repeat cycle q 21 to 28 days.*
or	carboplatin	Paraplatin	400 mg/m² I.V., day 1
	fluorouracil (5-FU)	Adrucil	1,000 mg/m² daily by continuous I.V. infusion, days 1 to 5 *Repeat cycle q 21 to 28 days.*
CFL (Head and neck cancer)	cisplatin	Platinol	100 mg/m² I.V., day 1
	fluorouracil (5-FU)	Adrucil	600 to 800 mg/m² daily by continuous I.V. infusion, days 1 to 5
	leucovorin calcium	Wellcovorin	200 to 300 mg/m² I.V. daily, days 1 to 5 *Repeat cycle q 21 days.*
CFM (Breast cancer)	cyclophosphamide	Cytoxan	500 mg/m² I.V., day 1
	fluorouracil (5-FU)	Adrucil	500 mg/m² I.V., day 1
	mitoxantrone	Novantrone	10 mg/m² I.V., day 1 *Repeat cycle q 21 days.*

(continued)

Cancer chemotherapy: Acronyms and protocols *(continued)*

ACRONYM AND INDICATION	DRUG		DOSAGE
	Generic name	Trade name	
CFPT (Breast cancer)	cyclophosphamide	Cytoxan	150 mg/m² I.V., days 1 to 5
	fluorouracil (5-FU)	Adrucil	300 mg/m² I.V., days 1 to 5
	prednisone	Deltasone	10 mg P.O. t.i.d. for first 7 days of each course
	tamoxifen	Nolvadex	10 mg P.O. b.i.d. (daily through each course) *Repeat cycle q 6 weeks.*
CHAP (Ovarian cancer, epithelial)	cyclophosphamide	Cytoxan	300 to 500 mg/m² I.V., day 1
	altretamine	Hexalen	150 mg/m² P.O., days 1 to 7
	doxorubicin	Adriamycin	30 to 50 mg/m² I.V., day 1
	cisplatin	Platinol	50 mg/m² I.V., day 1 *Repeat cycle q 28 days.*
ChIVPP (Hodgkin's lymphoma)	chlorambucil	Leukeran	6 mg/m² P.O., days 1 to 14 (10 mg/day maximum)
	vinblastine	Velban	6 mg/m² I.V., days 1 to 8 (10 mg/day maximum)
	procarbazine	Matulane	50 mg P.O., days 1 to 14 (150 mg/day maximum)
	prednisone	Deltasone	40 mg/m² P.O., days 1 to 14 (25 mg/m² for child)
CHOP (Non-Hodgkin's lymphoma)	cyclophosphamide	Cytoxan	750 mg/m² I.V., day 1
	doxorubicin	Adriamycin	50 mg/m² I.V., day 1
	vincristine	Oncovin	1.4 mg/m² (2 mg maximum) I.V., day 1
	prednisone	Deltasone	100 mg/m² P.O., days 1 to 5 *Repeat cycle q 21 days.*
CHOP-Bleo (Non-Hodgkin's lymphoma)	cyclophosphamide	Cytoxan	750 mg/m² I.V., day 1
	doxorubicin	Adriamycin	50 mg/m² I.V., day 1
	vincristine	Oncovin	2 mg I.V., days 1 and 5
	prednisone	Deltasone	100 mg P.O., days 1 to 5
	bleomycin	Blenoxane	15 units I.V., days 1 and 5 *Repeat cycle q 21 days.*
CISCA (Genitourinary cancer)	cyclophosphamide	Cytoxan	650 mg/m² I.V., day 1
	doxorubicin	Adriamycin	50 mg/m² I.V., day 1
	cisplatin	Platinol	70 to 100 mg/m² I.V., day 2 *Repeat cycle q 21 to 28 days.*

Cancer chemotherapy: Acronyms and protocols *(continued)*

ACRONYM AND INDICATION	DRUG		DOSAGE
	Generic name	Trade name	
CMF (Breast cancer)	cyclophosphamide	Cytoxan	100 mg/m² P.O., days 1 to 14, or 400 to 600 mg/m² I.V., day 1
	methotrexate	Folex	40 to 60 mg/m² I.V., days 1 and 8
	fluorouracil (5-FU)	Adrucil	400 to 600 mg/m² I.V., days 1 and 8 *Repeat cycle q 28 days.*
CMFVP (Cooper's) (Breast cancer)	cyclophosphamide	Cytoxan	2 to 2.5 mg/kg P.O. daily for 9 months
	methotrexate	Folex	0.7 mg/kg/week I.V. for 8 weeks, then every other week for 7 months
	fluorouracil (5-FU)	Adrucil	12 mg/kg/week I.V. for 8 weeks, then weekly for 7 months
	vincristine	Oncovin	0.035 mg/kg (2 mg/week maximum) I.V. for 5 weeks, then once monthly
	prednisone	Deltasone	0.75 mg/kg P.O. daily, days 1 to 10, then taper over next 40 days and discontinue
CMFVP (SWOG) (Breast cancer)	cyclophosphamide	Cytoxan	60 mg/m² P.O. daily for 1 year
	methotrexate	Folex	15 mg/m² I.V. weekly for 1 year
	fluorouracil (5-FU)	Adrucil	300 mg/m² I.V. weekly for 1 year
	vincristine	Oncovin	0.625 mg/m² I.V. weekly for 1 year
	prednisone	Deltasone	30 mg/m² P.O., days 1 to 14; 20 mg/m², days 15 to 28; 10 mg/m², days 29 to 42 *Repeat cycle q 42 days.*
COAP (Leukemia— AML, induction)	cyclophosphamide	Cytoxan	100 mg/m² I.V. or P.O., days 1 to 5
	vincristine	Oncovin	2 mg/m² I.V., day 1
	cytarabine (ara-C)	Cytosar-U	100 mg/m² I.V., days 1 to 5
	prednisone	Deltasone	100 mg P.O., days 1 to 5
COB (Head and neck cancer	cisplatin	Platinol	100 mg/m² I.V., day 1
	vincristine	Oncovin	1 mg I.V., days 2 and 5
	bleomycin	Blenoxane	30 units by continuous I.V. infusion, days 2 to 5 *Repeat cycle q 21 days.*

(continued)

Cancer chemotherapy: Acronyms and protocols *(continued)*

ACRONYM AND INDICATION	DRUG Generic name	Trade name	DOSAGE
COMLA (Non-Hodgkin's lymphoma)	cyclophosphamide	Cytoxan	1,500 mg/m² I.V., day 1
	vincristine	Oncovin	1.4 mg/m² (2.5 mg maximum) I.V., days 1, 8, and 15
	methotrexate	Folex	120 mg/m² I.V., days 22, 29, 36, 43, 50, 57, 64, and 71
	leucovorin calcium	Wellcovorin	25 mg/m² P.O. q 6 hours for four doses, beginning 24 hours after methotrexate dose
	cytarabine (ara-C)	Cytosar-U	300 mg/m² I.V., days 22, 29, 36, 43, 50, 57, 64, and 71 *Repeat cycle q 21 days.*
COP (Non-Hodgkin's lymphoma)	cyclophosphamide	Cytoxan	800 to 1,000 mg/m² I.V., day 1
	vincristine	Oncovin	1.4 mg/m² (2 mg maximum) I.V., day 1
	prednisone	Deltasone	60 mg/m² P.O., days 1 to 5 *Repeat cycle q 21 days.*
COP-BLAM (Non-Hodgkin's lymphoma)	cyclophosphamide	Cytoxan	400 mg/m² I.V., day 1
	vincristine	Oncovin	1 mg/m² I.V., day 1
	prednisone	Deltasone	40 mg/m² P.O., days 1 to 10
	bleomycin	Blenoxane	15 mg I.V., day 14
	doxorubicin	Adriamycin	40 mg/m², day 1
	procarbazine	Matulane	100 mg/m², days 1 to 10
COPE (Small-cell lung cancer)	cyclophosphamide	Cytoxan	750 mg/m² I.V., day 1
	cisplatin	Platinol	20 mg/m² I.V., days 1 to 3
	etoposide (VP-16)	VePesid	100 mg/m² I.V., days 1 to 3
	vincristine	Oncovin	2 mg/m² I.V., day 3 *Repeat cycle q 21 days.*
COPP (Non-Hodgkin's lymphoma)	cyclophosphamide	Cytoxan	400 to 650 mg/m² I.V., days 1 and 8
	vincristine	Oncovin	1.4 to 1.5 mg/m² (2 mg maximum) I.V., days 1 and 8
	procarbazine	Matulane	100 mg/m² P.O., days 1 to 10 or 1 to 14
	prednisone	Deltasone	40 mg/m² P.O., days 1 to 14 *Repeat cycle q 28 days.*
CP (Ovarian cancer, epithelial)	cyclophosphamide	Cytoxan	1,000 mg/m² I.V., day 1
	cisplatin	Platinol	50 to 60 mg/m² I.V., day 1 *Repeat cycle q 21 days.*

Cancer chemotherapy: Acronyms and protocols   *(continued)*

ACRONYM AND INDICATION	DRUG		DOSAGE
	Generic name	Trade name	
CV (Small-cell lung cancer)	cisplatin	Platinol	50 mg/m² I.V., day 1
	etoposide (VP-16)	VePesid	60 mg/m² I.V., days 1 to 5 *Repeat cycle q 21 to 28 days.*
CV (Non-small-cell lung cancer)	cisplatin	Platinol	60 to 80 mg/m² I.V., day 1
	etoposide (VP-16)	VePesid	120 mg/m² I.V., days 4, 6, and 8 *Repeat cycle q 21 to 28 days.*
CVEB (Genitourinary cancer)	cisplatin	Platinol	40 mg/m² I.V., days 1 to 5
	vinblastine	Velban	7.5 mg/m² I.V., day 1
	etoposide (VP-16)	VePesid	100 mg/m² I.V., days 1 to 5
	bleomycin	Blenoxane	30 units I.V. weekly *Repeat cycle q 21 days.*
CVI (VIC) (Non-small-cell lung cancer)	carboplatin	Paraplatin	300 mg/m² I.V., day 1
	etoposide (VP-16)	VePesid	60 to 100 mg/m² I.V., day 1
	ifosfamide	Ifex	1.5 g/m² I.V., days 1, 3, and 5
	mesna	Mesnex	Dosage is 20% of ifosfamide dose, given immediately before and at 4 and 8 hours after ifosfamide infusion *Repeat cycle q 28 days.*
CVP (Leukemia — CLL, blast crisis)	cyclophosphamide	Cytoxan	300 mg/m² P.O., days 1 to 5
	vincristine	Oncovin	1.4 mg/m² (2 mg maximum) I.V., day 1
	prednisone	Deltasone	100 mg/m² P.O., days 1 to 5 *Repeat cycle q 21 days.*
CVP (Non-Hodgkin's lymphoma)	cyclophosphamide	Cytoxan	400 mg/m² P.O., days 1 to 5
	vincristine	Oncovin	1.4 mg/m² (2 mg maximum) I.V., day 1
	prednisone	Deltasone	100 mg/m² P.O., days 1 to 5 *Repeat cycle q 21 days.*
CVPP (Hodgkin's lymphoma)	lomustine (CCNU)	CeeNU	75 mg/m² P.O., day 1
	vinblastine	Velban	4 mg/m² I.V., days 1 and 8
	procarbazine	Matulane	100 mg/m² P.O., days 1 to 14
	prednisone	Deltasone	30 mg/m² P.O., days 1 to 14 (cycles 1 and 4 only) *Repeat cycle q 28 days.*

(continued)

Cancer chemotherapy: Acronyms and protocols *(continued)*

ACRONYM AND INDICATION	DRUG		DOSAGE
	Generic name	Trade name	
CYADIC (Soft-tissue sarcoma)	cyclophosphamide	Cytoxan	600 mg/m² I.V., day 1
	doxorubicin	Adriamycin	15 mg/m² by continuous I.V. infusion, days 1 to 4
	dacarbazine	DTIC-Dome	250 mg/m² by continuous I.V. infusion, days 1 to 4
CYVADIC (Bony sarcoma)	cyclophosphamide	Cytoxan	600 mg/m² I.V., day 1
	vincristine	Oncovin	1.4 mg/m² (2 mg maximum) I.V. weekly for 6 weeks, then on day 1 of future cycles
	doxorubicin	Adriamycin	15 mg/m² by continuous I.V. infusion, days 1 to 4
	dacarbazine	DTIC-Dome	250 mg/m² by continuous I.V. infusion, days 1 to 4 *Repeat cycle q 21 to 28 days.*
CYVADIC (Soft-tissue sarcoma)	cyclophosphamide	Cytoxan	500 mg/m² I.V., day 1
	vincristine	Oncovin	1.4 mg/m² (2 mg maximum) I.V., days 1 and 5
	doxorubicin	Adriamycin	50 mg/m² I.V., day 1
	dacarbazine	DTIC-Dome	250 mg/m² I.V., days 1 to 5 *Repeat cycle q 21 days.*
DC (Leukemia— pediatric AML, induction)	daunorubicin	Cerubidine	45 to 60 mg/m² I.V., days 1 to 3
	cytarabine (ara-C)	Cytosar-U	100 mg/m² I.V. or S.C. q 12 hours for 5 to 7 days
DCPM (Leukemia— pediatric AML, induction)	daunorubicin	Cerubidine	25 mg/m² I.V., day 1
	cytarabine (ara-C)	Cytosar-U	80 mg/m² I.V., days 1 to 3
	prednisone	Deltasone	40 mg/m² P.O. daily
	mercaptopurine (6-MP)	Purinethol	100 mg/m² P.O. daily
DCT (Leukemia— ANLL, induction)	daunorubicin	Cerubidine	60 mg/m² I.V., days 1 to 3
	cytarabine (ara-C)	Cytosar-U	200 mg/m² daily by continuous I.V. infusion, days 1 to 5
	thioguanine (6-TG)		100 mg/m² P.O. q 12 hours, days 1 to 5
DHAP (Hodgkin's lymphoma)	dexamethasone	Decadron	40 mg P.O. or I.V., days 1 to 4
	cisplatin	Platinol	100 mg/m² by continuous I.V. infusion, day 1
	cytarabine (ara-C)	Cytosar-U	2 g/m² I.V. q 12 hours for two doses, day 2 *Repeat cycle q 3 to 4 weeks.*

Cancer chemotherapy: Acronyms and protocols *(continued)*

ACRONYM AND INDICATION	DRUG		DOSAGE
	Generic name	Trade name	
DTIC-ACTD (Malignant melanoma)	dacarbazine	DTIC-Dome	750 mg/m² I.V., day 1
	dactinomycin (actinomycin D)	Cosmegen	1 mg/m² I.V., day 1 *Repeat cycle q 28 days.*
DVP (Leukemia—ALL, induction)	daunorubicin	Cerubidine	45 mg/m² I.V., days 1 to 4
	vincristine	Oncovin	2 mg/m² (2 mg maximum) I.V. weekly for 4 weeks
	prednisone	Deltasone	45 mg/m² P.O., for 28 to 35 days
EP (Small-cell or non-small-cell lung cancer)	cisplatin	Platinol	75 to 100 mg/m² I.V., day 1
	etoposide (VP-16)	VePesid	75 to 100 mg/m² I.V., days 1 to 3 *Repeat cycle q 21 to 28 days.*
ESHAP (Non-Hodgkin's lymphoma)	etoposide (VP-16)	VePesid	40 mg/m² by continuous I.V. infusion, days 1 to 4
	cisplatin	Platinol	25 mg/m² daily by continuous I.V. infusion, days 1 to 4
	cytarabine (ara-C)	Cytosar-U	2 g/m² I.V. immediately after completion of etoposide and cisplatin therapy
	methylprednisolone	Solu-Medrol	500 mg I.V. daily, days 1 to 4 *Repeat cycle q 21 to 28 days.*
EVA (Hodgkin's lymphoma)	etoposide (VP-16)	VePesid	100 mg/m² I.V., days 1 to 3
	vinblastine	Velban	6 mg/m² I.V., day 1
	doxorubicin	Adriamycin	50 mg/m² I.V., day 1 *Repeat cycle q 28 days.*
FAC (CAF) (Breast cancer)	fluorouracil (5-FU)	Adrucil	500 mg/m² I.V., days 1 and 8
	doxorubicin	Adriamycin	50 mg/m² I.V., day 1
	cyclophosphamide	Cytoxan	500 mg/m² I.V., day 1 *Repeat cycle q 21 days.*
FAM (Colon cancer; gastric cancer)	fluorouracil (5-FU)	Adrucil	600 mg/m² I.V., days 1, 8, 29, and 36
	doxorubicin	Adriamycin	30 mg/m² I.V., days 1sion, days 2 to 6
	mitomycin	Mutamycin	10 mg/m² I.V., day 1 *Repeat cycle q 8 weeks.*
FAM (Non-small-cell lung cancer)	fluorouracil (5-FU)	Adrucil	600 mg/m² I.V., days 1, 8, 28, and 36
	doxorubicin	Adriamycin	30 mg/m² I.V., days 1 and 28
	mitomycin	Mutamycin	10 mg/m² I.V., day 1 *Repeat cycle q 8 weeks.*

(continued)

Cancer chemotherapy: Acronyms and protocols *(continued)*

ACRONYM AND INDICATION	DRUG		DOSAGE
	Generic name	Trade name	
FAM (Pancreatic cancer)	fluorouracil (5-FU)	Adrucil	600 mg/m² I.V., days 1, 8, 29, and 36
	doxorubicin	Adriamycin	30 mg/m² I.V., days 1 and 29
	mitomycin	Mutamycin	10 mg/m² I.V., day 1 *Repeat cycle q 8 weeks.*
FAME (Gastric cancer)	fluorouracil (5-FU)	Adrucil	350 mg/m² I.V., days 1 to 5 and 36 to 40
	doxorubicin	Adriamycin	40 mg/m² I.V., days 1 and 36
	semustine (methyl CCNU)		150 mg/m² P.O., day 1 *Repeat cycle q 10 weeks.*
FCE (Gastric cancer)	fluorouracil (5-FU)	Adrucil	900 mg/m² by continuous I.V. infusion, days 1 to 5
	cisplatin	Platinol	20 mg/m² I.V., days 1 to 5
	etoposide (VP-16)	VePesid	90 mg/m² I.V., days 1, 3, and 5 *Repeat cycle q 21 days.*
F-CL (Colon cancer)	fluorouracil (5-FU)	Adrucil	370 to 400 mg/m² I.V., days 1 to 5
	leucovorin calcium	Wellcovorin	200 mg/m² daily I.V., days 1 to 5, begun 15 minutes before fluorouracil infusion *Repeat cycle q 21 days.*
5 + 2 (Leukemia— ANLL, consolidation)	cytarabine (ara-C)	Cytosar-U	100 mg/m² I.V. q 12 hours for 6 days
	daunorubicin	Cerubidine	45 mg/m² I.V., days 1 and 2
FL (Genitourinary cancer) *or*	flutamide	Eulexin	250 mg P.O. t.i.d.
	leuprolide acetate	Lupron	1 mg S.C. daily
	flutamide	Eulexin	250 mg P.O. t.i.d.
	leuprolide acetate	Lupron Depot	7.5 mg I.M. q 28 days
FLe (Colon cancer)	levamisole	Ergamisol	50 mg P.O. t.i.d. for 3 days, repeated q 2 weeks for 1 year
	fluorouracil (5-FU)	Adrucil	450 mg/m² I.V. for 5 days, then, after a pause of 4 weeks, 450 mg/m² I.V. weekly for 48 weeks
FMS (Pancreatic cancer)	fluorouracil (5-FU)	Adrucil	600 mg/m² I.V., days 1, 8, 29, and 36
	mitomycin	Mutamycin	10 mg/m² I.V., day 1
	streptozocin	Zanosar	1 g/m² I.V., days 1, 8, 29, and 36 *Repeat cycle q 8 weeks.*

Cancer chemotherapy: Acronyms and protocols *(continued)*

ACRONYM AND INDICATION	DRUG		DOSAGE
	Generic name	Trade name	
FMV (Colon cancer)	fluorouracil (5-FU)	Adrucil	10 mg/kg I.V., days 1 to 5
	semustine (methyl CCNU)		175 mg/m² P.O., day 1
	vincristine	Oncovin	1 mg/m² (2 mg maximum) I.V., day 1 *Repeat cycle q 35 days.*
FZ (Genitourinary cancer)	flutamide	Eulexin	250 P.O. t.i.d.
	goserelin acetate	Zoladex	3.6 mg implant S.C. q 28 days
HDMTX (high-dose methotrexate) (Bony sarcoma)	methotrexate	Folex	12 g/m² I.V. (20 g maximum)
	leucovorin calcium	Wellcovorin	15 mg I.V. or P.O. q 6 hours for 10 doses, beginning 24 hours after methotrexate dose (serum methotrexate levels must be monitored) *Repeat cycle q 4 to 16 weeks.*
Hexa-CAF (Ovarian cancer, epithelial)	altretamine	Hexalen	150 mg/m² P.O., days 1 to 14
	cyclophosphamide	Cytoxan	150 mg/m² P.O., days 1 to 14
	methotrexate	Folex	40 mg/m², days 1 and 8
	fluorouracil (5-FU)	Adrucil	600 mg/m² I.V., days 1 and 8 *Repeat cycle q 28 days.*
HiDAC (Leukemia— ANLL, consolidation)	cytarabine (ara-C)	Cytosar-U	3,000 mg/m² I.V. q 12 hours, days 1 to 6
IMF (Breast cancer)	ifosfamide	Ifex	1.5 g/m² I.V., days 1 and 8
	mesna	Mesnex	Dosage is 20% of ifosfamide dose, given immediately before and at 4 and 8 hours after ifosfamide infusion
	methotrexate	Folex	40 mg/m² I.V., days 1 and 8
	fluorouracil (5-FU)	Adrucil	600 mg/m² I.V., days 1 and 8 *Repeat cycle q 28 days.*
L-VAM (Genitourinary cancer)	leuprolide acetate	Lupron	1 mg S.C. daily
	vinblastine	Velban	1.5 mg/m² by continuous I.V. infusion, days 2 to 7
	doxorubicin	Adriamycin	50 mg/m² by 24-hour continuous I.V. infusion, day 1
	mitomycin	Mutamycin	10 mg/m² I.V., day 2 *Repeat VAM cycle q 28 days.*

(continued)

Cancer chemotherapy: Acronyms and protocols *(continued)*

ACRONYM AND INDICATION	DRUG		DOSAGE
	Generic name	Trade name	
MACC (Non-small-cell lung cancer)	methotrexate	Folex	30 to 40 mg/m² I.V., day 1
	doxorubicin	Adriamycin	30 to 40 mg/m² I.V., day 1
	cyclophosphamide	Cytoxan	400 to 600 mg/m² I.V., day 1
	lomustine (CCNU)	CeeNU	30 to 40 mg/m² P.O., day 1 *Repeat cycle q 21 to 28 days.*
MACOP-B (Non-Hodgkin's lymphoma)	methotrexate	Folex	100 mg/m² I.V., weeks 2, 6, and 10; then 300 mg/m² I.V. for 4 hours, weeks 2, 6, and 10
	leucovorin calcium	Wellcovorin	15 mg P.O. q 6 hours for 6 doses, beginning 24 hours after methotrexate
	doxorubicin	Adriamycin	50 mg/m² I.V., weeks 1, 3, 5, 7, 9, and 11
	cyclophosphamide	Cytoxan	350 mg/m² I.V., weeks 1, 3, 5, 7, 9, and 11
	vincristine	Oncovin	1.4 mg/m² I.V. (2 mg maximum), weeks 2, 4, 8, 10, and 12
	bleomycin	Blenoxane	10 mg/m² I.V., weeks 4, 8, and 12
	prednisone	Deltasone	75 mg P.O. daily
MAID (Bony sarcoma)	mesna	Mesnex	Uroprotection 1.5 g/m² by continuous I.V. infusion, days 1 to 4
	doxorubicin	Adriamycin	15 mg/m² by continuous I.V. infusion, days 1 to 3
	ifosfamide	Ifex	1.5 g/m² by continuous I.V. infusion, days 1 to 3
	dacarbazine	DTIC-Dome	250 mg/m² by continuous I.V. infusion, days 1 to 3 *Repeat cycle q 21 to 28 days.*
MAID (Soft-tissue sarcoma)	mesna	Mesnex	1.5 g/m² by continuous I.V. infusion, days 1 to 4
	doxorubicin	Adriamycin	15 mg/m² by continuous I.V. infusion, days 1 to 3
	ifosfamide	Ifex	1.5 g/m² by continuous I.V. infusion, days 1 to 3
	dacarbazine	DTIC-Dome	250 mg/m² by continuous I.V. infusion, days 1 to 3 *Repeat cycle q 21 to 28 days.*
MAP (Head and neck cancer)	mitomycin	Mutamycin	8 mg/m² I.V., day 1
	doxorubicin	Adriamycin	40 mg/m² I.V., day 1
	cisplatin	Platinol	60 mg/m² I.V., day 1 *Repeat cycle q 28 days.*

Cancer chemotherapy: Acronyms and protocols *(continued)*

ACRONYM AND INDICATION	DRUG Generic name	Trade name	DOSAGE
m-BACOD (Non-Hodgkin's lymphoma)	bleomycin	Blenoxane	4 units/m² I.V., day 1
	doxorubicin	Adriamycin	45 mg/m² I.V., day 1
	cyclophosphamide	Cytoxan	600 mg/m² I.V., day 1
	vincristine	Oncovin	1 mg/m² I.V., day 1
	dexamethasone	Decadron	6 mg/m² I.V., days 1 to 5
	methotrexate	Folex	200 mg/m² I.V., days 8 and 15
	leucovorin calcium	Wellcovorin	10 mg/m² P.O. q 6 hours for 8 doses, beginning 24 hours after methotrexate dose *Repeat cycle q 21 days.*
m-BACOS (Non-Hodgkin's lymphoma)	doxorubicin	Adriamycin	50 mg/m² by 24-hour continuous I.V. infusion, day 1
	vincristine	Oncovin	1.4 mg/m² (2 mg maximum) I.V., day 1
	bleomycin	Blenoxane	10 units/m² I.V., day 1
	cyclophosphamide	Cytoxan	750 mg/m² I.V., day 1
	methotrexate	Folex	1 g/m² I.V., day 2
	leucovorin calcium	Wellcovorin	15 mg P.O. q 6 hours for 8 doses starting 24 hours after methotrexate dose *Repeat cycle q 21 to 25 days.*
MBC (Head and neck cancer)	methotrexate	Folex	40 mg/m² I.M. or I.V., days 1 and 15
	bleomycin	Blenoxane	10 units I.M. or I.V. weekly
	cisplatin	Platinol	50 mg/m² I.V., day 1 *Repeat cycle q 21 days.*
MC (Leukemia— ANLL, consolidation)	mitoxantrone	Novantrone	12 mg/m² I.V. daily, days 1 and 2
	cytarabine (ara-C)	Cytosar-U	100 mg/m² daily by continuous I.V. infusion, days 1 to 5 *Repeat cycle.*
MC (Leukemia— ANLL, induction)	mitoxantrone	Novantrone	12 mg/m² I.V., days 1 to 3 and 17 to 18
	cytarabine (ara-C)	Cytosar-U	100 mg/m² daily by continuous I.V. infusion, days 1 to 7 and 17 to 21
MF (Head and neck cancer)	methotrexate	Folex	125 to 150 mg/m² I.V., day 1
	fluorouracil (5-FU)	Adrucil	600 mg/m² I.V., beginning 1 hour after methotrexate dose
	leucovorin calcium	Wellcovorin	10 mg/m² I.V. or P.O. q 6 hours for 5 doses, beginning 24 hours after methotrexate dose *Repeat cycle weekly.*

(continued)

Cancer chemotherapy: Acronyms and protocols *(continued)*

ACRONYM AND INDICATION	DRUG Generic name	Trade name	DOSAGE
MICE (ICE) (Small-cell and non-small-cell lung cancer)	mesna	Mesnex	Dosage is 20% of ifosfamide doses given I.V. immediately before and at 4 and 8 hours after ifosfamide infusion
	ifosfamide	Ifex	2,000 mg/m² I.V., days 1 to 3
	carboplatin	Paraplatin	300 to 350 mg/m² I.V., day 1
	etoposide (VP-16)	VePesid	60 to 100 mg/m² I.V., days 1 to 3
MINE (Non-Hodgkin's lymphoma)	mesna	Mesnex	1.3 to 1.5 g/m² I.V., days 1 to 3
	ifosfamide	Ifex	1.3 to 1.5 g/m² I.V., days 1 to 3
	mitoxantrone	Novantrone	8 to 10 mg/m² I.V., day 1
	etoposide (VP-16)	VePesid	65 to 80 mg/m² I.V., days 1 to 3
MM (Leukemia — ALL, maintenance)	mercaptopurine (6-MP)	Purinethol	50 mg/m² P.O. daily
	methotrexate	Folex	20 mg/m² P.O. or I.V. weekly
MOF (Colon cancer)	fluorouracil (5-FU)	Adrucil	10 mg/kg/day I.V., days 1 to 5
	semustine (methyl CCNU)		175 mg/m² P.O., day 1
	vincristine	Oncovin	1 mg/m² (2 mg maximum) I.V., day 1 *Repeat cycle q 35 days.*
MOP (Pediatric brain tumors)	mechlorethamine (nitrogen mustard)	Mustargen	6 mg/m² I.V., days 1 and 8
	vincristine	Oncovin	1.4 mg/m² (2 mg maximum) I.V., days 1 and 8
	procarbazine	Matulane	100 mg/m² P.O., days 1 to 14 *Repeat cycle q 28 days.*
MOPP (Hodgkin's lymphoma)	mechlorethamine (nitrogen mustard)	Mustargen	6 mg/m² I.V., days 1 and 8
	vincristine	Oncovin	1.4 mg/m² (2 mg maximum) I.V., days 1 and 8
	procarbazine	Matulane	100 mg/m² P.O., days 1 to 14
	prednisone	Deltasone	40 mg/m² P.O., days 1 to 14 *Repeat cycle q 28 days.*
MP (Multiple myeloma)	melphalan (L-phenylalanine mustard)	Alkeran	8 mg/m² P.O., days 1 to 4
	prednisone	Deltasone	40 mg/m² P.O., days 1 to 7 *Repeat cycle q 28 days.*

Cancer chemotherapy: Acronyms and protocols *(continued)*

ACRONYM AND INDICATION	DRUG		DOSAGE
	Generic name	Trade name	
m-PFL (Genitourinary cancer)	methotrexate	Folex	60 mg/m², day 1
	cisplatin	Platinol	25 mg/m² by continuous I.V. infusion, days 2 to 6
	fluorouracil (5-FU)	Adrucil	800 mg/m² by continuous I.V. infusion, days 2 to 6
	leucovorin calcium	Wellcovorin	500 mg/m² by continuous I.V. infusion, days 2 to 6 *Repeat cycle q 28 days for four cycles.*
M-2 (Multiple myeloma)	vincristine	Oncovin	0.03 mg/kg (2 mg maximum) I.V., day 1
	carmustine	BiCNU	0.5 mg/kg I.V., day 1
	cyclophosphamide	Cytoxan	10 mg/kg I.V, day 1
	melphalan (L-phenylalanine mustard)	Alkeran	0.25 mg/kg P.O., days 1 to 14
	prednisone	Deltasone	1 mg/kg, days 1 to 7, then taper over next 14 days *Repeat cycle q 35 days.*
MV (Leukemia— AML, induction)	mitoxantrone	Novantrone	10 mg/m² I.V., days 1 to 5
	etoposide (VP-16)	VePesid	100 mg/m² I.V., days 1 to 3
MVAC (Genitourinary cancer)	methotrexate	Folex	30 mg/m² I.V., days 1, 15, and 22
	vinblastine	Velban	3 mg/m² I.V., days 2, 15, and 22
	doxorubicin	Adriamycin	30 mg/m² I.V., day 2
	cisplatin	Platinol	70 mg/m² I.V., day 2 *Repeat cycle q 28 days.*
MVP (Non-small-cell lung cancer)	mitomycin	Mutamycin	8 mg/m² I.V., days 1, 29, and 71
	vinblastine	Velban	4.5 mg/m² I.V., days 15, 22, and 29, then q 2 weeks
	cisplatin	Platinol	120 mg/m² I.V., days 1 and 29, then q 6 weeks
MVPP (Hodgkin's lymphoma)	mechlorethamine (nitrogen mustard)	Mustargen	6 mg/m² I.V., days 1 and 8
	vinblastine	Velban	6 mg/m² I.V., days 1 and 8
	procarbazine	Matulane	100 mg/m² P.O., days 1 to 14
	prednisone	Deltasone	40 mg/m² P.O., days 1 to 14 *Repeat cycle q 42 days for six cycles.*

(continued)

Cancer chemotherapy: Acronyms and protocols *(continued)*

ACRONYM AND INDICATION	DRUG		DOSAGE
	Generic name	Trade name	
OPEN (Non-Hodgkin's lymphoma)	vincristine	Oncovin	2 mg I.V., day 1
	prednisone	Deltasone	100 mg P.O. daily for 5 days
	etoposide (VP-16)	VePesid	100 mg/m² I.V. daily for 3 days
	mitoxantrone	Novantrone	10 mg/m² I.V., day 1
PCV (Pediatric brain tumors)	procarbazine	Matulane	60 mg/m² P.O., days 18 to 21
	lomustine (CCNU)	CeeNU	110 mg/m² P.O., day 1
	vincristine	Oncovin	1.4 mg/m² (2 mg maximum), days 8 and 29 *Repeat cycle q 6 to 8 weeks.*
PFL (Head and neck cancer)	cisplatin	Platinol	25 mg/m² by continuous I.V. infusion, days 1 to 5
	fluorouracil (5-FU)	Adrucil	800 mg/m² by continuous I.V. infusion, days 2 to 6
	leucovorin calcium	Wellcovorin	500 mg/m² by continuous I.V. infusion, days 1 to 6 *Repeat cycle q 28 days.*
PFL (Non-small-cell lung cancer)	cisplatin	Platinol	25 mg/m² I.V., days 1 and 15
	fluorouracil (5-FU)	Adrucil	800 mg/m² by continuous I.V. infusion, days 1 to 5
	leucovorin calcium	Wellcovorin	500 mg/m² by continuous I.V. infusion, days 1 to 5 *Repeat cycle q 28 days.*
ProMACE (Non-Hodgkin's lymphoma)	prednisone	Deltasone	60 mg/m² P.O., days 1 to 14
	methotrexate	Folex	1.5 g/m² I.V., day 14
	leucovorin calcium	Wellcovorin	50 mg/m² I.V. q 6 hours for 5 doses, beginning 24 hours after methotrexate dose
	doxorubicin	Adriamycin	25 mg/m² I.V., days 1 and 8
	cyclophosphamide	Cytoxan	650 mg/m² I.V., days 1 and 8
	etoposide (VP-16)	VePesid	120 mg/m² I.V., days 1 and 8 *Repeat cycle q 28 days; MOPP therapy to begin after the required number of ProMACE cycles are completed.*

Cancer chemotherapy: Acronyms and protocols *(continued)*

ACRONYM AND INDICATION	DRUG		DOSAGE
	Generic name	Trade name	
ProMACE/ cytaBOM (Non-Hodgkin's lymphoma)	cyclophosphamide	Cytoxan	650 mg/m² I.V., day 1
	doxorubicin	Adriamycin	25 mg/m² I.V., day 1
	etoposide (VP-16)	VePesid	120 mg/m² I.V., day 1
	prednisone	Deltasone	60 mg/m² P.O., days 1 to 14
	cytarabine (ara-C)	Cytosar-U	300 mg/m² I.V., day 8
	bleomycin	Blenoxane	5 mg/m² I.V., day 8
	vincristine	Oncovin	1.4 mg/m² I.V., day 8
	methotrexate	Folex	120 mg/m² I.V., day 8
	leucovorin calcium	Wellcovorin	25 mg/m² P.O. q 6 hours for 4 doses *Repeat cycle q 28 days.*
(pulse) VAC (Soft-tissue sarcoma)	vincristine	Oncovin	1.5 g/m² (2 mg maximum) I.V., day 1 or weekly, starting on day 1
	dactinomycin (actinomycin D)	Cosmegen	0.4 mg/m² I.V., day 1
	cyclophosphamide	Cytoxan	1,000 mg/m² I.V., day 1 *Repeat cycle q 3 to 4 weeks.*
7 + 3 (A + D) (Leukemia— AML, induction)	cytarabine (ara-C)	Cytosar-U	100 or 200 mg/m² by continuous I.V. infusion, days 1 to 7
	daunorubicin	Cerubidine	45 mg/m² I.V., days 1 to 3
TC (Leukemia— ANLL, maintenance)	thioguanine (6-TG)		40 mg/m² P.O. q 12 hours for 8 doses, days 1 to 4
	cytarabine (ara-C)	Cytosar-U	60 mg/m² S.C. day 5 *Repeat cycle weekly.*
T-10 (Pediatric bony sarcoma)	methotrexate	Folex	12 g/m² I.V. for 12 or 16 doses
	leucovorin calcium	Wellcovorin	15 mg I.V. or P.O. q 6 hours for 10 doses, each starting 20 hours after methotrexate dose
	doxorubicin	Adriamycin	30 mg/m² I.V. for 2 to 3 days
	cisplatin	Platinol	120 mg/m² I.V. for 1 day
	bleomycin	Blenoxane	15 units/m² I.V. for 2 days
	cyclophosphamide	Cytoxan	600 mg/m² I.V. for 2 days
	dactinomycin (actinomycin D)	Cosmegen	0.6 mg/m² I.V. for 2 days

(continued)

Cancer chemotherapy: Acronyms and protocols (continued)

ACRONYM AND INDICATION	DRUG		DOSAGE
	Generic name	Trade name	
VA (Wilms' tumor)	vincristine	Oncovin	1.5 mg/m² (2 mg maximum) weekly
	dactinomycin (actinomycin D)	Cosmegen	0.4 mg/m² q 2 weeks
VAB (Genitourinary cancer)	vinblastine	Velban	4 mg/m² I.V., day 1
	dactinomycin (actinomycin D)	Cosmegen	1 mg/m² I.V., day 1
	bleomycin	Blenoxane	30 units I.V. push, then 20 units/m² by continuous I.V. infusion, days 1 to 3
	cisplatin	Platinol	120 mg/m² I.V., day 4
	cyclophosphamide	Cytoxan	600 mg/m² I.V., day 1 *Repeat cycle q 21 days.*
VAC (Small-cell lung cancer)	vincristine	Oncovin	2 mg I.V., day 1
	doxorubicin	Adriamycin	50 mg/m² I.V., day 1
	cyclophosphamide	Cytoxan	750 mg/m² I.V., day 1 *Repeat cycle q 21 days for four cycles.*
VAC (Ovarian cancer, germ-cell)	vincristine	Oncovin	1.2 to 1.5 mg/m² (2 mg maximum) I.V. weekly for 10 to 12 weeks, or q 2 weeks for 12 doses
	dactinomycin (actinomycin D)	Cosmegen	0.3 to 0.4 mg/m² I.V., days 1 to 5
	cyclophosphamide	Cytoxan	150 mg/m² I.V., days 1 to 5 *Repeat cycle q 28 days.*
VAC (Wilms' tumor)	vincristine	Oncovin	1.5 mg/m² (2 mg maximum) weekly
	dactinomycin (actinomycin D)	Cosmegen	1.25 g/m² q 3 weeks
	cyclophosphamide	Cytoxan	1,000 mg/m² q 3 weeks
VAD (Multiple myeloma)	vincristine	Oncovin	0.4 mg by continuous I.V. infusion, days 1 to 4
	doxorubicin	Adriamycin	9 to 10 mg/m² by continuous I.V. infusion, days 1 to 4
	dexamethasone	Decadron	40 mg P.O. on days 1 to 4, 9 to 12, and 17 to 20 *Repeat cycle q 25 to 35 days.*

Cancer chemotherapy: Acronyms and protocols *(continued)*

ACRONYM AND INDICATION	DRUG		DOSAGE
	Generic name	Trade name	
VAP (VP + A) (Leukemia— pediatric ALL, induction)	vincristine	Oncovin	1.5 to 2 mg/m² (2 mg maximum) I.V. weekly for 4 weeks
	asparaginase	Elspar	10,000 units I.M., days 1 and 8 (other doses include 6,000 units/m² I.M. for 3 days/week or 25,000 units/m²)
	prednisone	Deltasone	40 mg/m² P.O., days 1 to 28, then taper over 7 days
VATH (Breast cancer)	vinblastine	Velban	4.5 mg/m² I.V., day 1
	doxorubicin	Adriamycin	45 mg/m² I.V., day 1
	thiotepa	Thiotepa	12 mg/m² I.V., day 1
	fluoxymesterone	Halotestin	30 mg P.O. (daily through each course) *Repeat cycle q 21 days.*
VB (Genitourinary cancer)	vinblastine	Velban	3 to 4 mg/m² I.V., day 1
	methotrexate	Folex	30 to 40 mg/m² I.V., day 1 *Repeat cycle weekly.*
VBAP (Multiple myeloma)	vincristine	Oncovin	1 mg I.V., day 1
	carmustine	BiCNU	30 mg/m² I.V., day 1
	doxorubicin	Adriamycin	30 mg/m² I.V., day 1
	prednisone	Deltasone	100 mg P.O., days 1 to 4 *Repeat cycle q 21 days.*
VBC (Malignant melanoma)	vinblastine	Velban	6 mg/m² I.V., days 1 and 2
	bleomycin	Blenoxane	15 units/m² by continuous I.V. infusion, days 1 to 5
	cisplatin	Platinol	50 mg/m² I.V., day 5 *Repeat cycle q 28 days.*
VBP (Genitourinary cancer)	vinblastine	Velban	6 mg/m² I.V., days 1 and 2
	bleomycin	Blenoxane	30 units I.V. weekly
	cisplatin	Platinol	20 mg/m² I.V., days 1 to 5 *Repeat cycle q 21 to 28 days.*
VC (Small-cell lung cancer)	etoposide (VP-16)	VePesid	100 to 200 mg/m² I.V., days 1 to 3
	carboplatin	Paraplatin	50 to 125 mg/m² I.V., days 1 to 3 *Repeat cycle q 28 days.*

(continued)

Cancer chemotherapy: Acronyms and protocols *(continued)*

ACRONYM AND INDICATION	DRUG		DOSAGE
	Generic name	Trade name	
VCAP (Multiple myeloma)	vincristine	Oncovin	1 mg I.V., day 1
	cyclophosphamide	Cytoxan	100 mg/m² P.O., days 1 to 4
	doxorubicin	Adriamycin	25 mg/m² I.V., day 2
	prednisone	Deltasone	60 mg/m² P.O., days 1 to 4 *Repeat cycle q 28 days.*
VDP (Malignant melanoma)	vinblastine	Velban	5 mg/m² I.V., days 1 and 2
	dacarbazine	DTIC-Dome	150 mg/m² I.V., days 1 to 5
	cisplatin	Platinol	75 mg/m² I.V., day 5 *Repeat cycle q 21 to 28 days.*
VIP (Genitourinary cancer)	vinblastine	Velban	0.11 mg/kg I.V., days 1 and 2
	ifosfamide	Ifex	1.2 g/m² I.V., days 1 to 5
	cisplatin	Platinol	20 mg/m², days 1 to 5
	mesna	Mesnex	400 mg I.V., 15 minutes before ifosfamide, then 1.2 g by continuous I.V. infusion, days 1 to 5 *Repeat cycle q 3 weeks for four cycles.*
or	etoposide (VP-16)	VePesid	75 mg/m² I.V., days 1 to 5
	ifosfamide	Ifex	1.2 g/m² I.V., days 1 to 5
	cisplatin	Platinol	20 mg/m², days 1 to 5
	mesna	Mesnex	400 mg I.V., 15 minutes before ifosfamide, then 1.2 g by continuous I.V. infusion, days 1 to 5 *Repeat cycle q 3 weeks for four cycles.*

Estimating body surface area in children

Pediatric drug dosages should be calculated on the basis of body surface area or body weight. To estimate a child's body surface area using this nomogram, place a straightedge on the correct height and weight points for your patient, and observe the point where it intersects on the surface area scale at center. *Note:* Don't use drug dosages based on body surface area in premature or full-term newborns. Instead, use body weight.

Nomogram

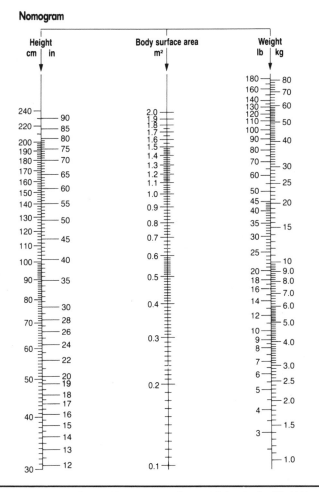

Reproduced from *Nelson Textbook of Pediatrics*, 14th ed. Courtesy W.B. Saunders Co., Philadelphia.

Estimating body surface area in adults

Place a straightedge from the patient's height in the left-hand column to his weight in the right-hand column. The intersection of this line with the center scale reveals the body surface area. The adult nomogram is especially useful in calculating dosages for chemotherapy.

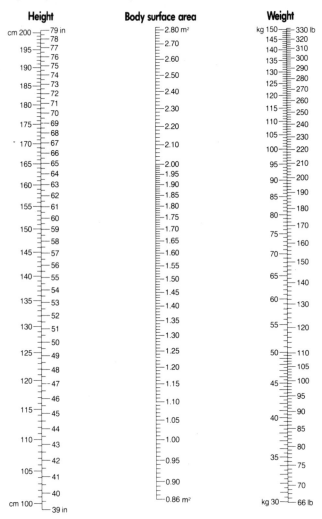

Calculating body surface area

$$BSA\ (m^2) = \sqrt{\frac{height \times weight}{3600}}$$

From Mostellar, R.D. "Simplified Calculation of Body-Surface Area," *New England Journal of Medicine* 317(17):1098, October 22, 1987.

$$BSA\ (m^2) = (wt^{0.425}) \times (ht^{0.725}) \times .007184$$

From Du Bois, D., and Du Bois, E. "A Formula to Estimate the Approximate Surface Area If Height and Weight Be Known," *Archives of Internal Medicine* 17:836-871, 1916.

$$BSA\ (m^2) = (wt^{0.5378}) \times (ht^{0.3964}) \times 0.024265$$

From Haycock, G.B., et. al. "Geometric Method for Measuring Body Surface Area: A Height-Weight Formula Validated in Infants, Children, and Adults," *Journal of Pediatrics* 93(1):62-66, July 1978.

BSA = body surface area; m^2 = meters squared; ht = height in centimeters; wt = weight in kilograms

Calculating body surface area in adult amputees

BODY PART	WOMEN (%)	MEN (%)
Hand plus 5 fingers	2.65	2.83
Lower part of arm	3.80	4.04
Upper part of arm	5.65	5.94
Foot	2.94	3.15
Lower part of leg	6.27	5.99
Thigh	12.55	11.80

$$BSA\ (M^2) = BSA - [(BSA \times \%\ BSA\ part)]$$

BSA = body surface area; M^2 = meters squared; BSA part = body surface area of amputated body part

Note: Dose reductions may not be necessary because metabolism and clearance of a drug dose do not necessarily change in adult amputees. Use professional judgment when deciding to reduce drug doses. (From Colangelo, P.M., et al. "Two Methods for Estimating Body Surface Area in Adult Amputees," *American Journal of Hospital Pharmacy* 41(21):2650-2655, December 1984.)

Controlling side effects of chemotherapy

Dear Patient:
Your doctor has ordered chemotherapy to treat your cancer. Besides treating cancer, these therapies often cause unpleasant side effects. Fortunately, you can sometimes prevent them. Other times you can do things to make yourself more comfortable. Just follow the advice below.

Mouth sores
• Keep your mouth and teeth clean by brushing after every meal with a soft toothbrush.
• Don't use commercial mouthwashes that contain alcohol, which may irritate your mouth during chemotherapy. Instead, rinse with water or water mixed with baking soda or use a suspension of sucralfate (Carafate) if your doctor orders it. Floss daily, and apply fluoride if your dentist recommends it. If you have dentures, be sure to remove them often for cleaning.
• Until your mouth sores heal, avoid foods that are difficult to chew (such as apples) or irritating to your mouth (such as acidic citrus juices). Also avoid drinking alcohol, smoking, and eating extremely hot or spicy foods.
• Eat soft, bland foods, such as eggs and oatmeal, and soothing foods, such as ice pops. Your doctor might also prescribe medication for mouth sores.

Dry mouth
• Frequently sip cool liquids and suck on ice chips or sugarless candy.
• Ask your doctor about artificial saliva. Use water, juices, sauces, and dressings to soften your food and make it easier to swallow. Don't smoke or drink alcohol, which can further dry your mouth.

Nausea and vomiting
• Before a chemotherapy treatment, try eating a light, bland snack, such as toast or crackers. Or don't eat anything—some patients find that fasting controls nausea better.
• Keep unpleasant odors out of your dining area. Avoid strong-smelling foods. Also brush your teeth before eating to refresh your mouth.
• Eat small, frequent meals and avoid lying down for 2 hours after you eat. Try small amounts of clear, unsweetened liquids, such as apple juice, and then progress to crackers or dry toast. Stay away from sweets and fried or other high-fat foods. It's best to stay with bland foods.
• Take antiemetic drugs, as your doctor orders. Be sure to notify him if vomiting is severe or lasts longer than 24 hours or if you urinate less, feel weak, or have a dry mouth.

Diarrhea
• Stick with low-fiber foods, such as bananas, rice, applesauce, toast, or mashed potatoes. Stay away from high-fiber foods, such as raw vegetables and fruits and whole-grain breads. Also avoid milk products and fruit juices. Cabbage, coffee, beans, and sweets can increase stomach cramps.

Controlling side effects of chemotherapy (continued)

- Because potassium may be lost when you have diarrhea, eat high-potassium foods, such as bananas and potatoes. Check with your doctor to see if you need a potassium supplement.
- After a bowel movement, clean your anal area gently and apply petroleum jelly (Vaseline) to prevent soreness.
- Ask your doctor about antidiarrheal medications. Notify him if your diarrhea doesn't stop or if you urinate less, have a dry mouth, or feel weak.

Constipation
- Eat high-fiber foods unless your doctor tells you otherwise. They include raw fruits and vegetables (with skins on, washed well), whole-grain breads and cereals, and beans. If you're not used to eating high-fiber foods, start gradually to let your body get accustomed to the change – or else you could develop diarrhea.
- Drink plenty of liquids – unless your doctor tells you not to.
- If changing your diet doesn't help, ask your doctor about stool softeners or laxatives. Check with your doctor before using enemas.

Heartburn
- Avoid spicy foods, alcohol, and smoking. Eat small, frequent meals.
- After eating, don't lie down right away. Avoid bending or stooping.
- Take oral medications with a glass of milk or a snack.
- Use antacids, as your doctor orders.

Muscle aches or pain, weakness, numbness or tingling
- Take acetaminophen (Tylenol). Or ask your doctor for acetaminophen with codeine.
- Apply heat where it hurts or feels numb.
- Be sure to rest. Also, avoid activities that aggravate your symptoms.
- If symptoms don't go away and pain focuses on one area, notify your doctor.

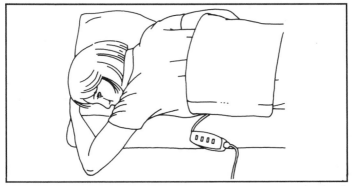

(continued)

Controlling side effects of chemotherapy *(continued)*

Hair loss
- Wash your hair gently. Use a mild shampoo and avoid frequent brushing or combing.
- Get a short haircut to make thinning hair less noticeable.
- Consider wearing a wig or toupee during therapy. Buy one before chemotherapy begins. Or use a hat, scarf, or turban to cover your head during therapy.

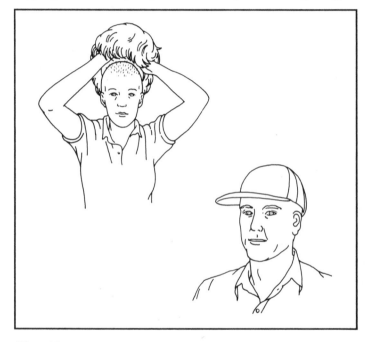

Skin problems
- For sensitive or dry skin, ask your doctor or nurse to recommend a lotion.
- Use cornstarch to absorb moisture, and avoid tight clothing over the treatment area. Be sure to report any blisters or cracked skin to the doctor.
- Stay out of the sun during the course of therapy. You may even have to avoid the sun for several months afterward, so check with your doctor, especially if you're planning a vacation to a sunny area. When you *can* go out in the sun

Controlling side effects of chemotherapy *(continued)*

again, wear light clothes over the treated area, and wear a hat, too. Cover all exposed skin with a good sun block lotion (skin protection factor [SPF] 15 or above).

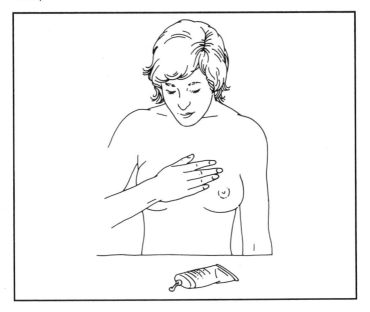

Tiredness
• Limit activities, especially sports.
• Get more sleep.
• Try to reduce your work hours until the end of treatments. Discuss your therapy schedule with your employer.
• If at all possible, schedule chemotherapy treatments at your convenience.
• Ask for help from family and friends, whether it's pitching in with daily chores or driving you to the hospital. Most people are glad to help out—they just need to be asked.
• If you lose interest in sex during treatments, either because you're too tired or because of hormonal changes, bear in mind that sexual desire usually returns after treatments end.

(continued)

Controlling side effects of chemotherapy *(continued)*

Risk of infection
You're more likely to get an infection during therapy, so follow these tips:
• Avoid crowds and people with colds and infections.
• Use an electric shaver instead of a razor.
• Use a soft toothbrush. It will help you avoid injuring your gums — a frequent site of infection.
• Tell your doctor if you have a fever, chills, a tendency to bruise easily, or any unusual bleeding.

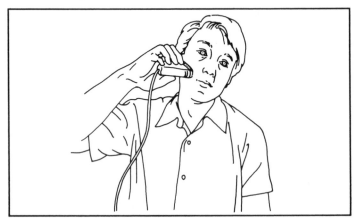

Additional instructions

_____

_____

_____

_____

_____

_____

Adding fiber to your diet

Dear Patient:
Here are four easy ways to add fiber to your diet.

Eat whole-grain breads and cereals
For the first few days, eat one serving daily of whole-grain breads (1 slice), cereal (½ cup), pasta (½ cup), or brown rice (⅓ cup). Examples of whole-grain breads are whole wheat and pumpernickel. Examples of high-fiber cereals are bran or oat flakes and shredded wheat. Gradually increase to four or more servings daily.

Eat fresh fruits and vegetables
Begin by eating one serving daily of raw or cooked, unpeeled fruit (one medium-size piece; ½ cup cooked) or unpeeled vegetables (½ cup cooked; 1 cup raw). Gradually increase to four servings daily. Examples of high-fiber fruits include apples, oranges, and peaches. Some high-fiber vegetables are carrots, corn, and peas.

Eat dried peas and beans
Begin by eating one serving (⅓ cup) a week. Increase to at least two to three servings a week.

Eat unprocessed bran
Add bran to your food. Start with 1 teaspoon a day, and over a 3-week period work up to 2 to 3 tablespoons a day. Don't use more than this. Remember to drink at least six 8-ounce (oz) glasses of fluid a day.

A small amount of bran can be beneficial, but too much can irritate your digestive tract, cause gas, interfere with mineral absorption, and even lodge in your intestine.

Note: Crisp fresh fruits and vegetables, cooked foods with husks, and nuts must be chewed thoroughly so that large particles don't pass whole into the intestine and lodge there, causing problems.

A sample menu

Breakfast
½ grapefruit
Oatmeal with milk and raisins (add bran if desired)
Bran muffin
8 oz liquid

(continued)

Adding fiber to your diet *(continued)*

Lunch
Cabbage slaw
Tuna salad sandwich on whole-wheat bread
Fresh pear with skin
8 oz liquid

Dinner
Vegetable soup
Broiled fish with almond topping
Baked potato with skin
Carrots and peas
Canned crushed pineapple
8 oz liquid

Snack
Dried fruit and nut mix
8 oz liquid

Additional instructions

_____

_____

_____

_____

_____

_____

_____

_____

_____

Stimulating your appetite

Dear Patient:
Your loss of appetite is a common side effect of cancer and its treatment. Try the following tips to stimulate your appetite.

Make mealtime more enjoyable
• Create a pleasant dining atmosphere. Accompany meals with music, soft lights, a brightly colored table setting, or whatever makes you feel good while eating. If permitted, have a glass of wine or beer with your meal to increase your appetite.
• Arrange food attractively on the plate. Add a garnish, such as parsley or a slice of lemon, to make the food appealing.
• Share meals with your family or friends. Or try watching television or reading while you eat.
• Eat frequent, small meals instead of three large meals.
• Keep nutritious snacks on hand — nuts, fruit, and cheese, for example — and eat whenever you feel hungry.

Be creative with your cooking
• Vary your diet and try new recipes. Experiment with spices and seasonings to make food more flavorful.
• If you can tolerate dairy products, add margarine or butter to foods to improve flavor. Also try mixing canned cream soups with milk rather than water, and adding cream sauce or melted cheese to vegetables.
• Drink milk shakes, eggnog, or prepared liquid food supplements between meals. You may want to enrich some beverages with eggs, honey, or powdered milk.

Overcome obstacles to eating
• Take a walk or exercise moderately before meals to help build your appetite.
• If nausea discourages you from eating, try to curb it by eating low-fat meals. Avoid overly sweet or spicy foods. Eat dry foods, such as toast or crackers, when you get up in the morning.
• Minimize mouth soreness or dryness by avoiding foods that are very salty, spicy, or hot. Instead, eat cold foods, such as ice cream, frozen yogurt, milk shakes, and cold soups. Ice chips, flavored ice pops, hard candies, lemon slices, and dill pickles help keep your mouth moist.
• If you live alone, consider contacting Meals On Wheels or a similar community program when you don't feel like cooking.

Adding calories to your diet

Dear Patient:
Here are some tips to help add calories to your diet.

Eat high-calorie snacks
Good choices include dried fruits, such as raisins and apricots; peanut butter or cheese spread on crackers, bread, fresh fruit, or raw vegetables; milk shakes made with ice cream, cream, powdered milk, or instant breakfast powders; and breakfast bars.

Add fat and sugar to food
• Put margarine or butter on bread, rice, noodles, potatoes, and vegetables. Use mayonnaise or margarine on sandwiches.
• Add sour cream to casseroles, or serve it with potatoes, vegetables, meat, and fruit.
• Serve meat, vegetables, and casseroles with cream sauces or gravy.
• Mix extra amounts of salad dressing in salads.
• Add whipped cream to hot chocolate, fruit, and desserts.
• Top ice cream with syrup or preserves.
• Spread bread, muffins, biscuits, or crackers with jam, jelly, or honey.
• Substitute half-and-half or cream for milk in coffee or tea.
• Add cheese to scrambled eggs, sauces, vegetables, casseroles, and salads.
• Use extra eggs in sauces, casseroles, sandwich spreads, and salads. Add powdered eggs to milk shakes. (Don't use raw eggs—they can cause food poisoning.)
• Sprinkle chopped or ground nuts on ice cream, yogurt, frozen yogurt, pudding, breads, and desserts. (Children under age 4 shouldn't eat whole nuts because they might choke.)

Use high-calorie supplements
If you've experienced lung damage, repeated infections, or weight loss, try adding commercial, high-protein calorie supplements to your daily diet. Typical commercial supplements include Ensure, Ensure Plus, Meritene, and Sustacal. Or use instant breakfast powders mixed with whole milk to get about the same number of calories and nutritional value as the supplements.

Additional instructions

Avoiding infection

Dear Patient:
As your doctor has explained, you have an increased risk of getting an infection. Here are some simple steps you can take to protect yourself.

Follow your doctor's directions
• Take all medications exactly as prescribed. Don't stop taking your medication unless directed by your doctor.
• Keep all medical appointments so that your doctor can monitor your progress and the drug's effects.
• If you're receiving a medication that puts you at risk for infection, be sure to tell your dentist or other doctors.

Minimize your exposure to infection
• Avoid crowds and people who have colds, flu, chicken pox, shingles, or other contagious illnesses.
• Don't receive any immunizations without checking with your doctor, especially live-virus vaccines, such as poliovirus vaccines. These contain weakened but living viruses that can cause illness in anyone who's taking a medication that puts him at risk for infection. Avoid contact with anyone who has recently been vaccinated.
• Practice good personal hygiene, especially hand washing.
• Before preparing food, wash your hands thoroughly. To avoid ingesting harmful organisms, thoroughly wash and cook all food before you eat it.
• Practice good oral hygiene.
• Don't use commercial mouthwashes because their high alcohol and sugar content may irritate your mouth and provide a medium for bacterial growth.
• Don't use unprescribed intravenous drugs – or at least don't share needles.
• If you travel to foreign countries, consider drinking only bottled or boiled water and avoiding raw vegetables and fruits to prevent a possible intestinal infection.
• Wear a mask and gloves to clean bird cages, fish tanks, or cat litter boxes.
• Keep rooms clean and well ventilated. Keep air conditioners and humidifiers cleaned and repaired so they don't harbor infectious organisms.

More prevention tips
• Get adequate sleep at night, and rest often during the day.
• Eat small, frequent meals, even if you've lost your appetite and have to force yourself to eat.

(continued)

Avoiding infection *(continued)*

Recognize symptoms of infection
Contact your doctor immediately or seek medical treatment for:
• persistent fever or nighttime sweating not related to a cold or the flu
• profound, persistent fatigue unrelieved by rest and not related to increased physical activity, longer work schedules, drug use, or a psychological disorder
• loss of appetite and weight loss
• open sores or ulcerations
• dry, persistent, unproductive cough
• persistent, unexplained diarrhea
• a white coating or spots on your tongue or throat, possibly with soreness, burning, or difficulty swallowing
• blurred vision or persistent, severe headaches
• confusion, depression, uncontrolled excitement, or inappropriate speech
• persistent or spreading rash or skin discoloration
• unexplained bleeding or bruising.

Washing your hands correctly

Dear Patient:
Everyday activities, such as petting your dog or sorting money, leave unwanted germs on your hands. These germs may enter your body and cause an infection. To prevent this, wash your hands several times daily — and always before meals. Here's how.

1 Wet your hands under lots of running water. This carries away contaminants.

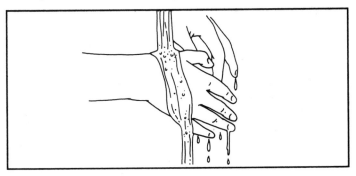

2 Lather your hands and wrists with soap. Although soap and water don't actually kill germs, they do loosen the skin oils and deposits that harbor germs. While you're washing, give your fingernails a good scrub, too.

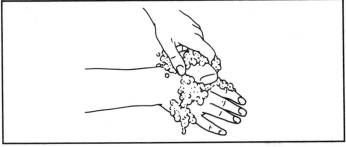

(continued)

Washing your hands correctly *(continued)*

3 Now, thoroughly rinse your hands in running water. Make sure your fingers point downward. That way runoff water won't travel up your arms to bring new germs down to your hands.

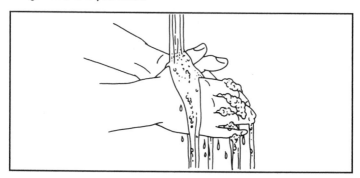

4 If you're at home, dry your hands with a clean cloth or paper towel. Don't dry off with a used towel, which may put germs right back on your hands. If you're in a public place, a hot-air hand dryer is best, but clean paper towels will do.

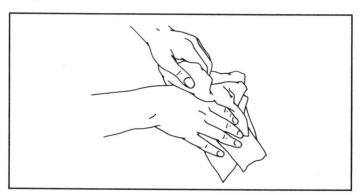

Help for dry hands
If your hands become dry or scratchy from frequent hand washing, soothe them with a hand lotion. And don't use strong soaps. They aren't needed for good hygiene, and they may cause drying or even allergic reactions.

Learning about bladder-instilled chemotherapy

Dear Patient:

The doctor will treat your bladder cancer by instilling medication directly into your bladder. This procedure is called intravesical chemotherapy.

Read the information below to learn what you can expect during your chemotherapy treatments. If you have questions, ask your nurse or doctor for more information.

How does the medication get into my bladder?

The medication reaches your bladder through a very thin tube called a catheter. The catheter will be inserted in your urethra, which is the opening through which you urinate. First, the urethra will be cleaned with a bacteria-fighting solution, such as povidone-iodine. Then the catheter will be inserted, and the urine that's already in your bladder will be drained into a container. Now, you should be ready to receive your treatment medication.

Next, the medication will be instilled through the catheter, and the catheter will remain in place for a certain period of time. During that time, the catheter will be clamped shut so that no medication can escape from the bladder.

Meanwhile, you may be asked to change your position by turning from side to side or walking around. This distributes the medication throughout your bladder.

How is the medication removed?

At the end of the scheduled time, the clamp on the catheter will be released, and the medication will drain out. Then the catheter will be removed. You shouldn't feel any discomfort while this is being done. Try to relax and take a few deep breaths. Afterward, you may wash your genital area.

What about side effects?

The side effects depend on the kind of medication you receive. For example:
• If you're receiving *triethylenethiophosphoramide* (also called Thiotepa), common side effects include fever, chills, a sore throat, hives, itching, bladder spasms, and pain when you urinate.
• If you're receiving *doxorubicin* (also called Adriamycin), you may have pain when you urinate, the sensation of having an urgent need to urinate, and discolored (cherry red) urine.
• If you're receiving *mitomycin* (also called Mutamycin), side effects include pain when you urinate, the sensation of having an urgent need to urinate, and a rash on your palms and buttocks.
• If you're receiving *bacillus Calmette-Guérin* (also called BCG), you may experience pain when you urinate, bladder spasms, blood in your urine, fever, chills, and muscle and joint aches.

Ask your doctor, nurse, or infusion therapist how best to relieve these side effects.

INDEX

i refers to an illustration; t refers to a table

i refers to an illustration; t refers to a table

i refers to an illustration; t refers to a table

i refers to an illustration; t refers to a table

i refers to an illustration; t refers to a table

i refers to an illustration; t refers to a table